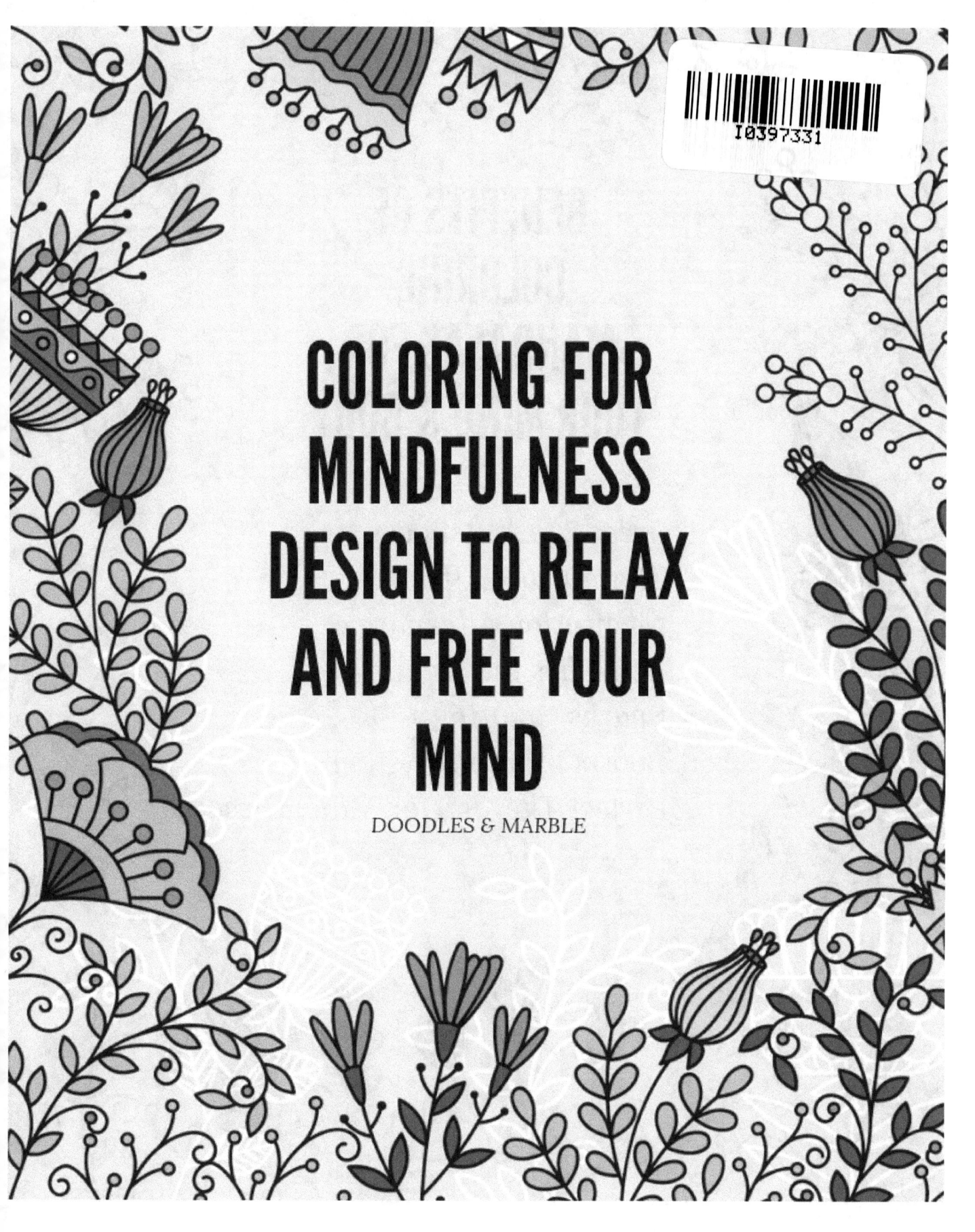

BENEFITS OF COLORING MANDALAS FOR YOUR MIND & BODY

DOODLES & MARBLE

1. Great Stress Reliever
2. Therapeutic Effect
3. Meditation Alternative
4. Refreshes the Brain
5. Sparks Creativity
6. Boosts Immune System
7. Perfect Therapy for Many Diseases

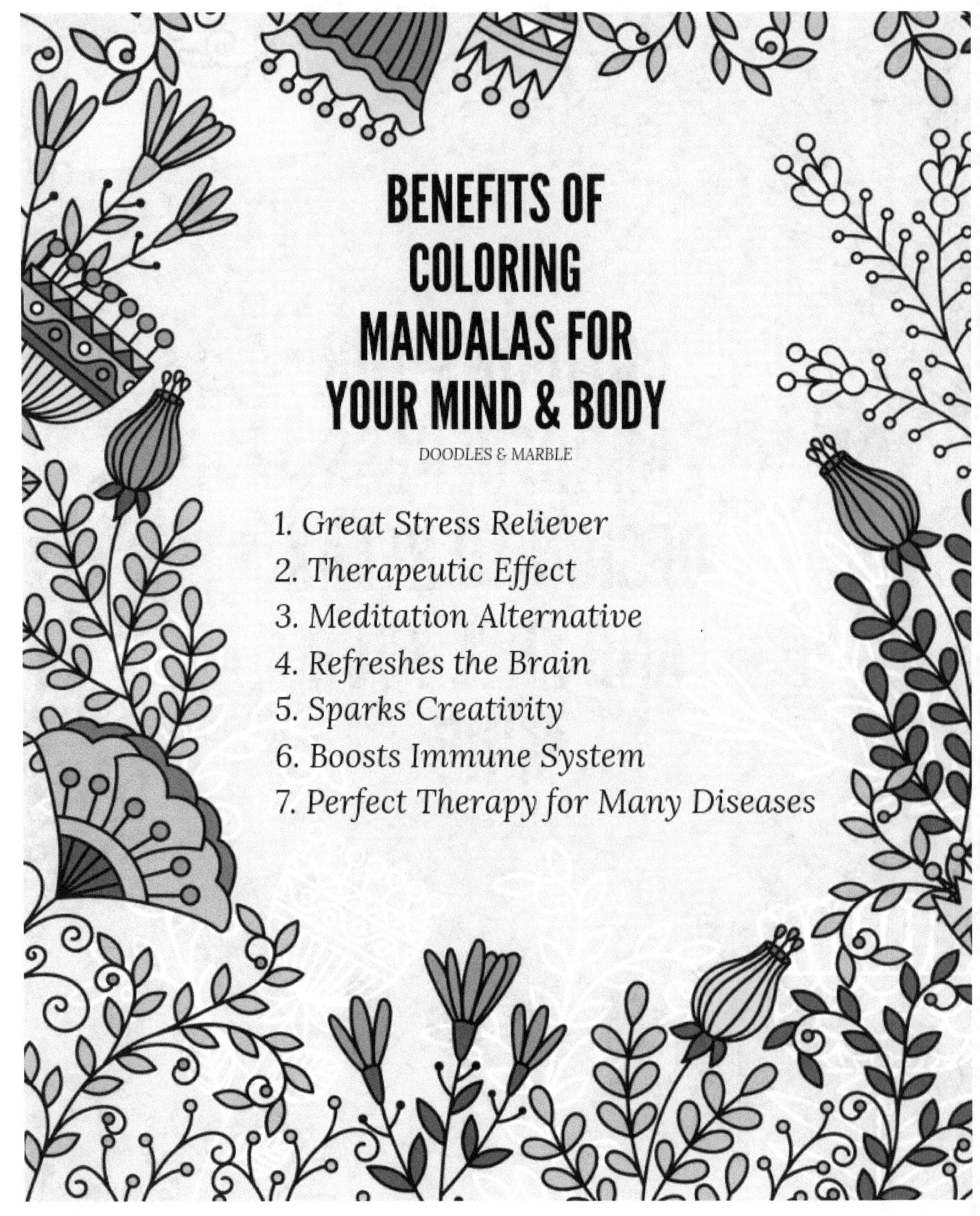

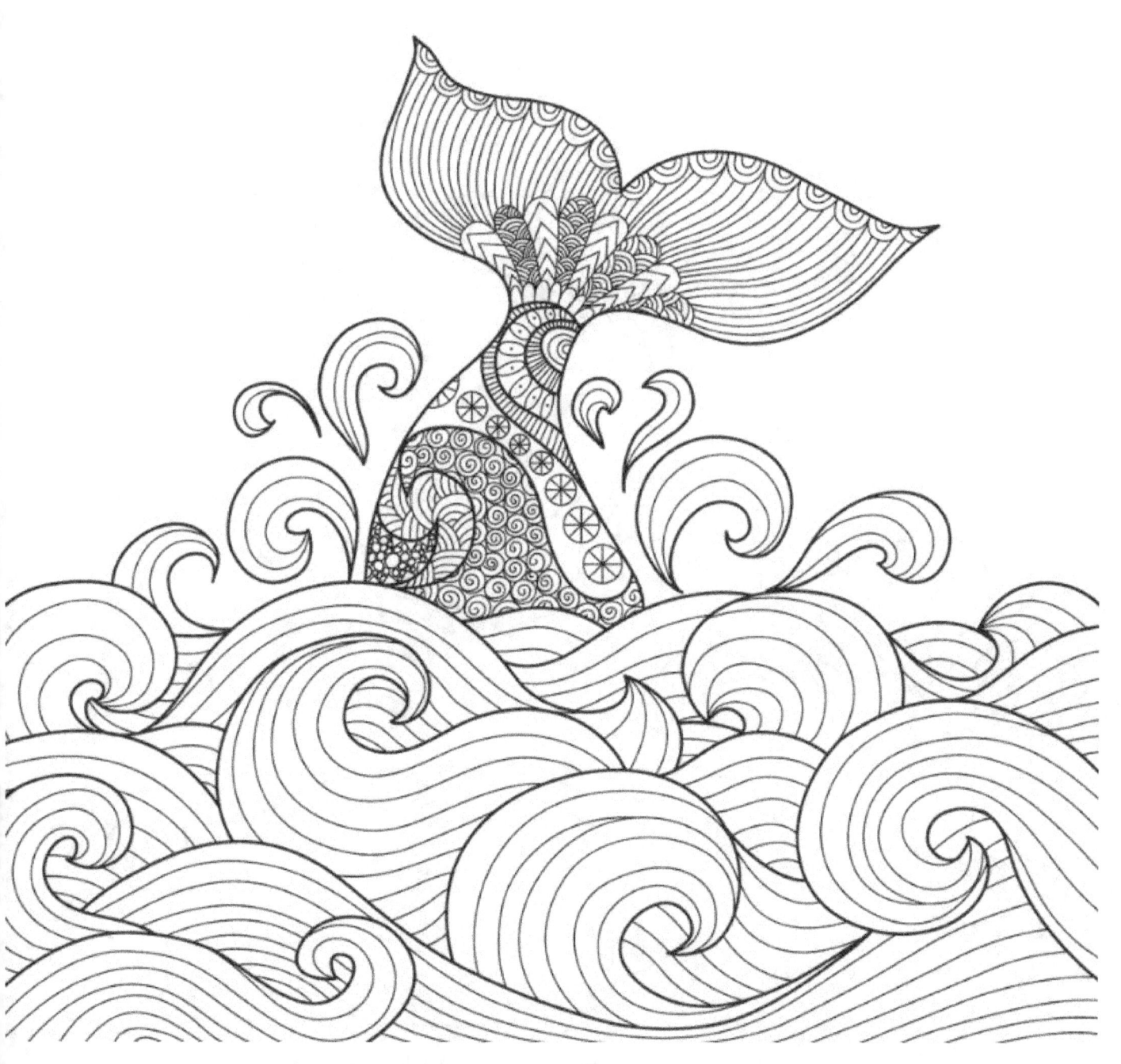

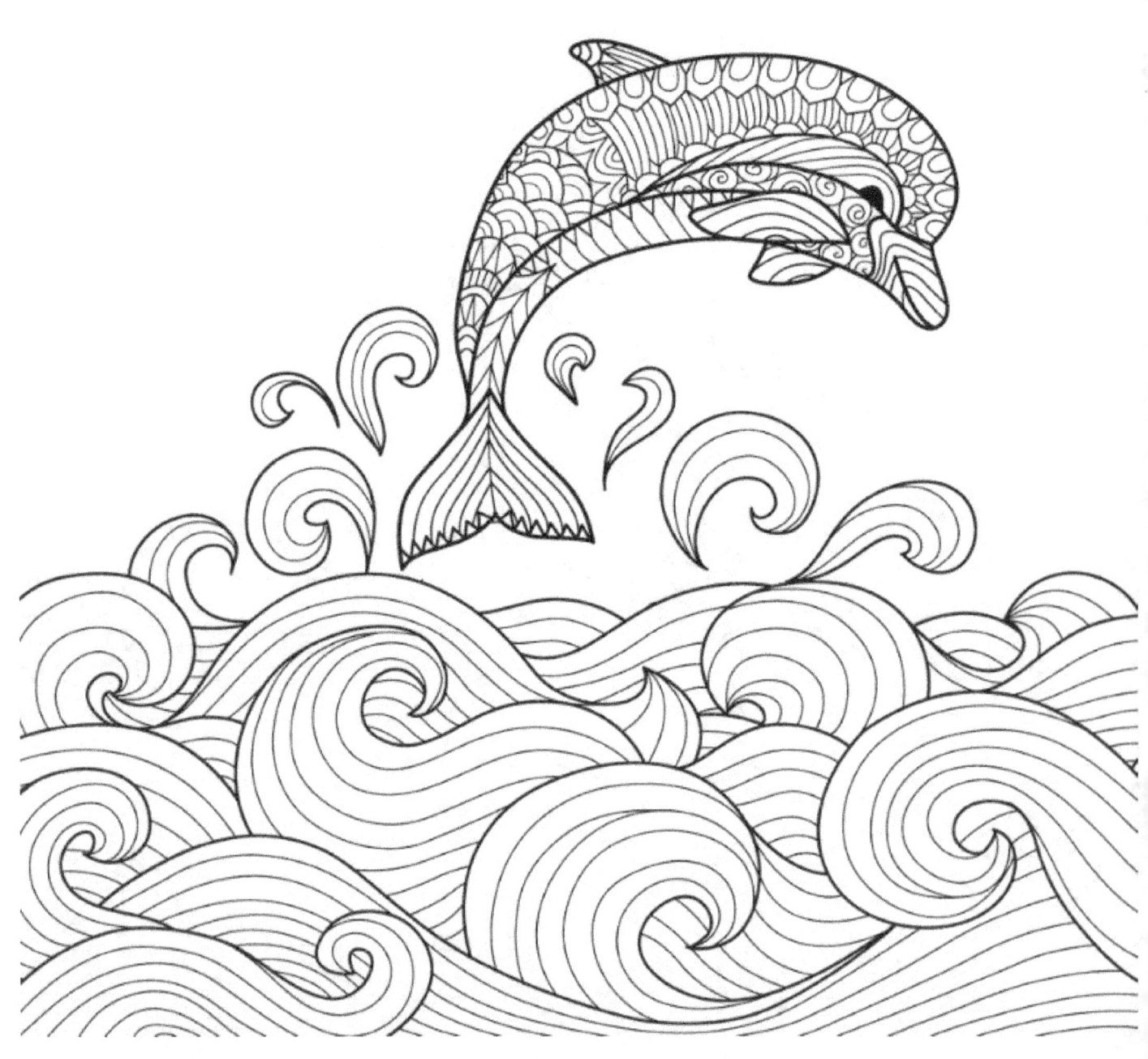

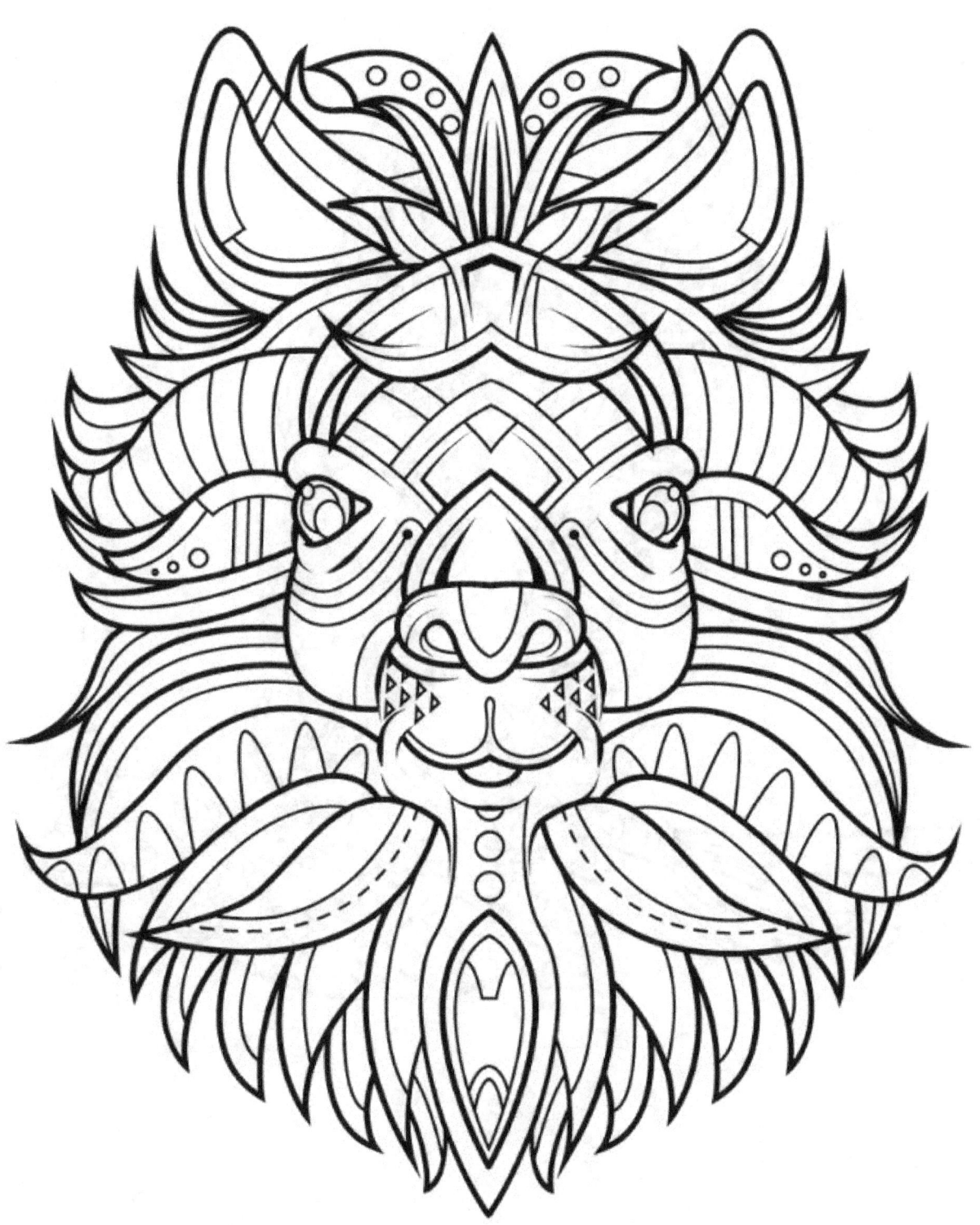

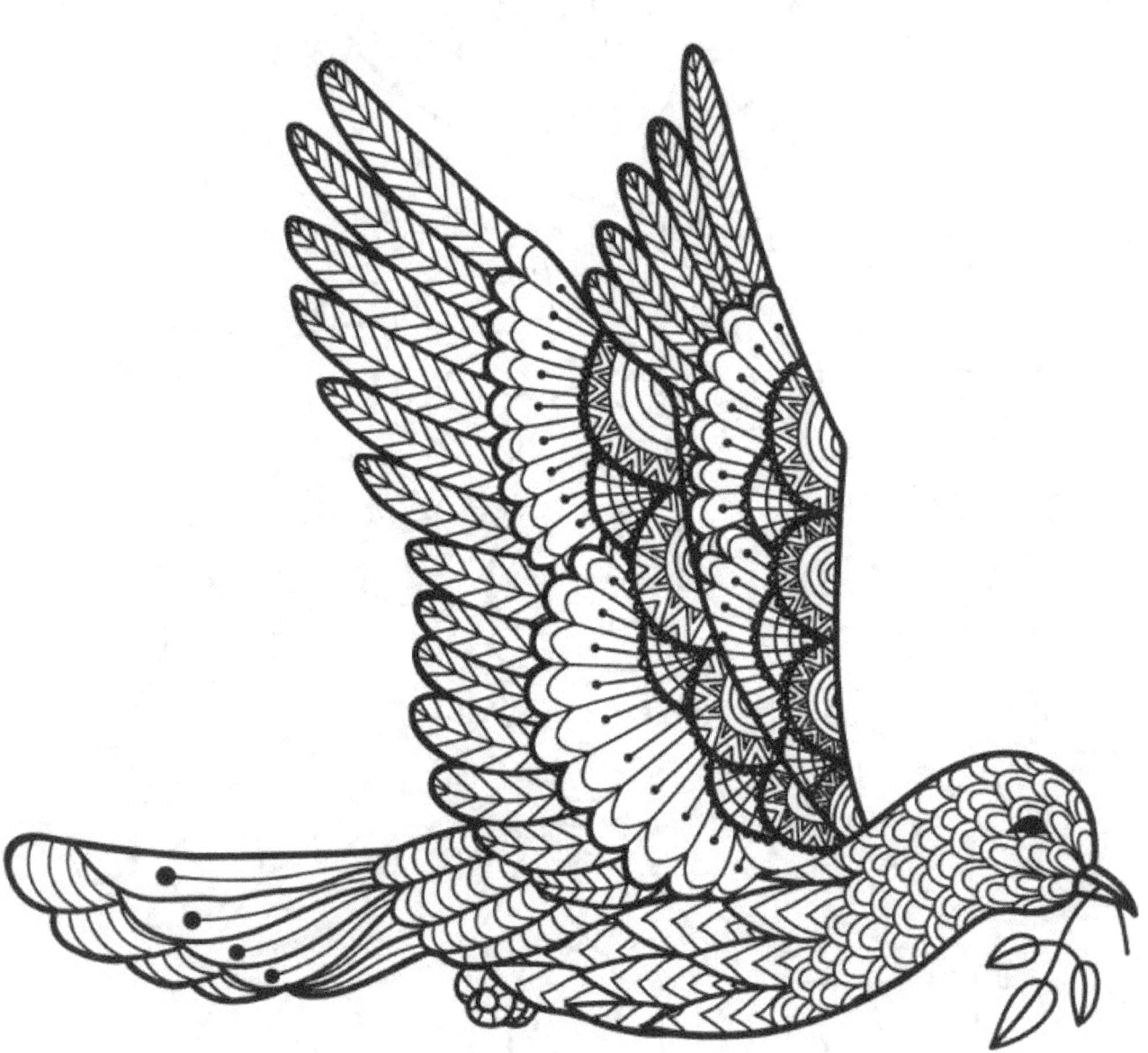

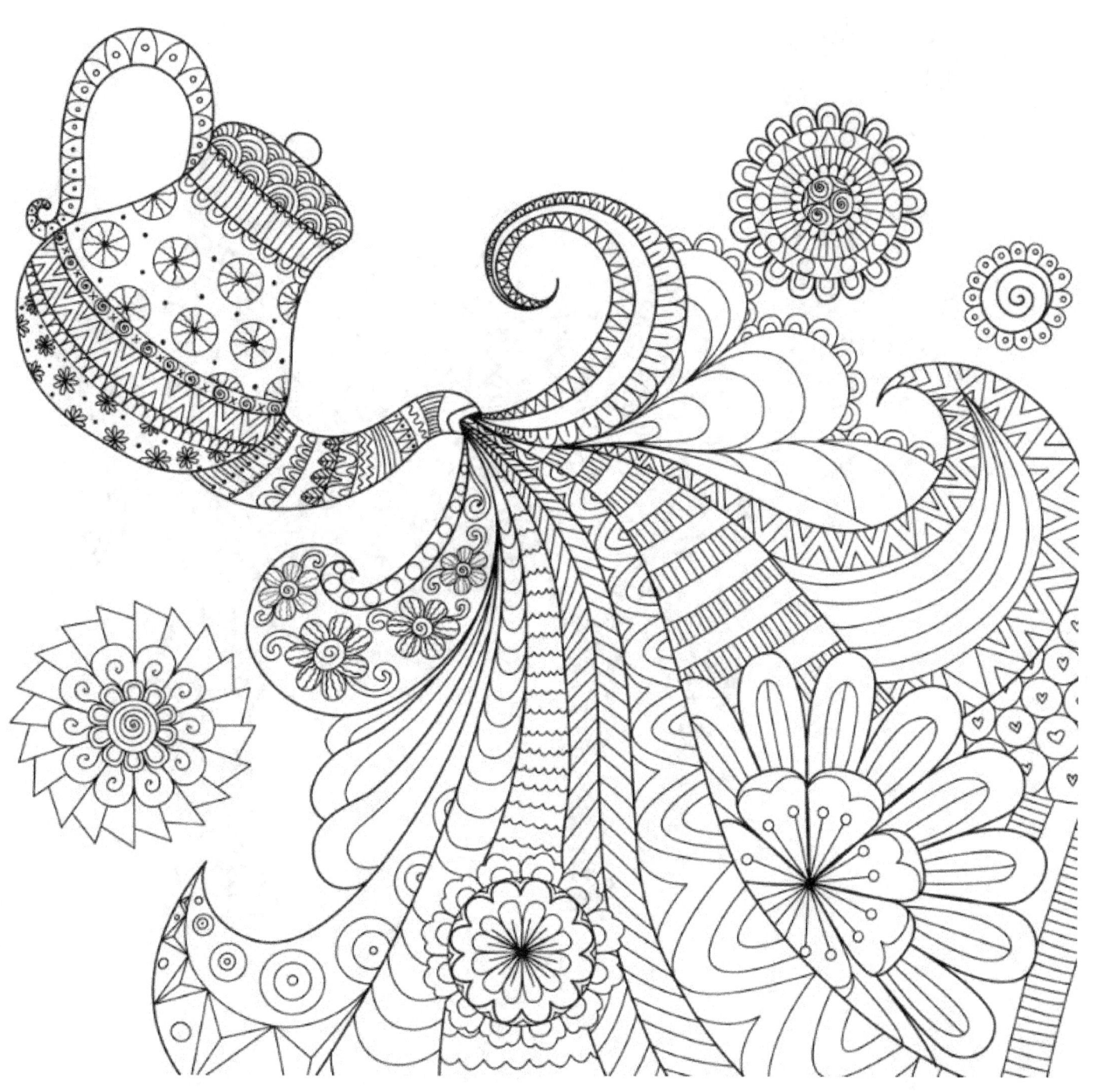

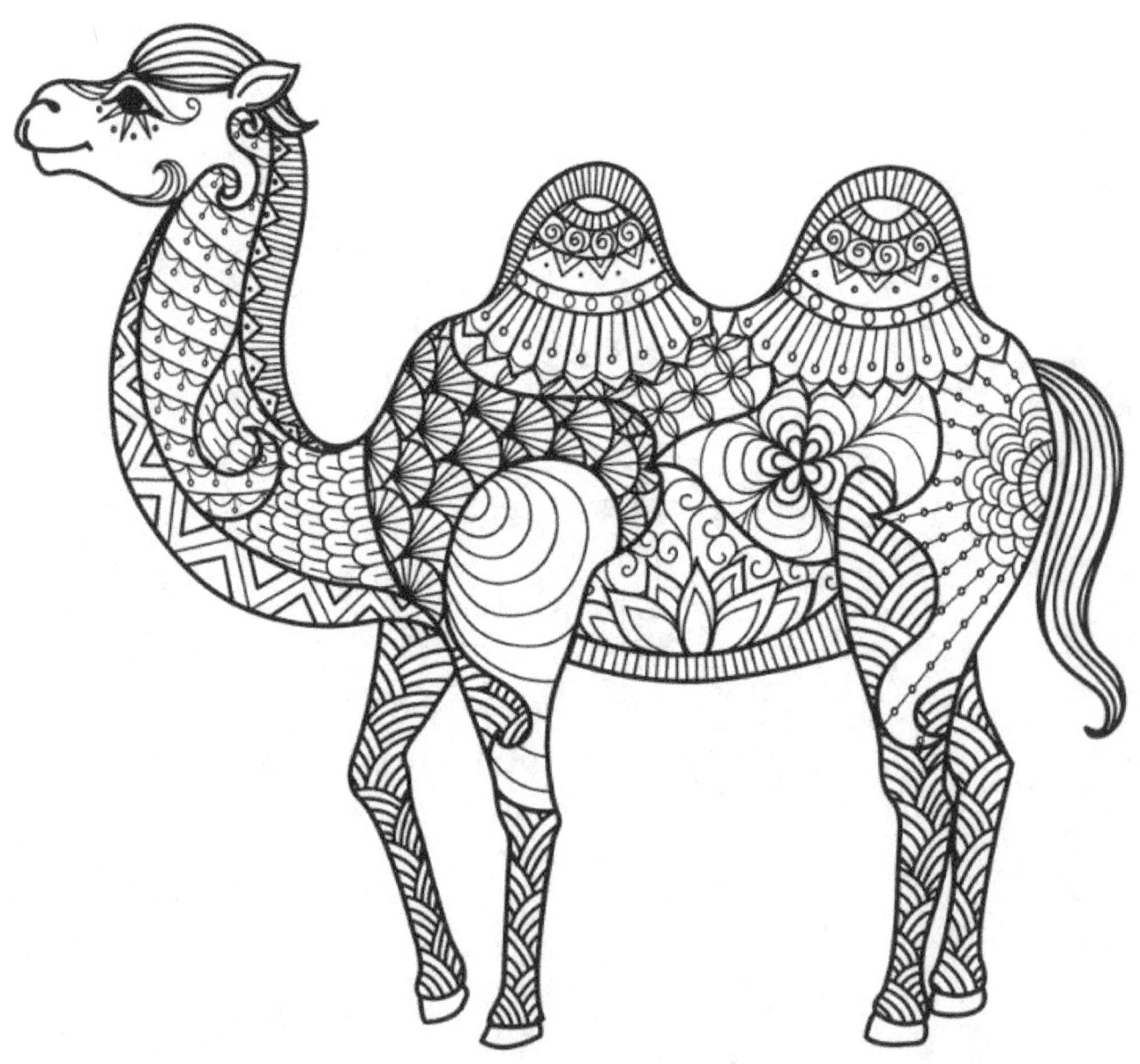

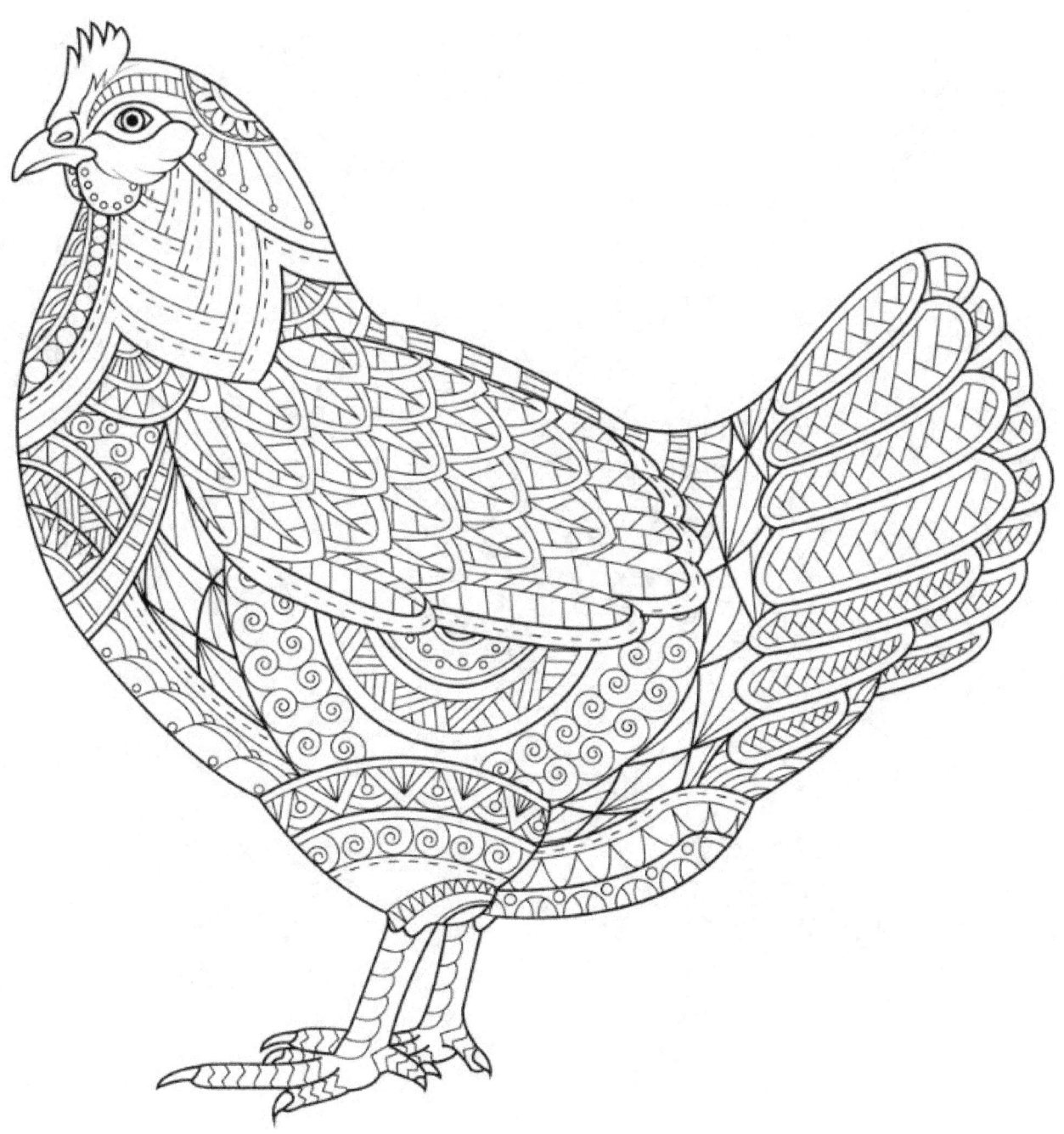

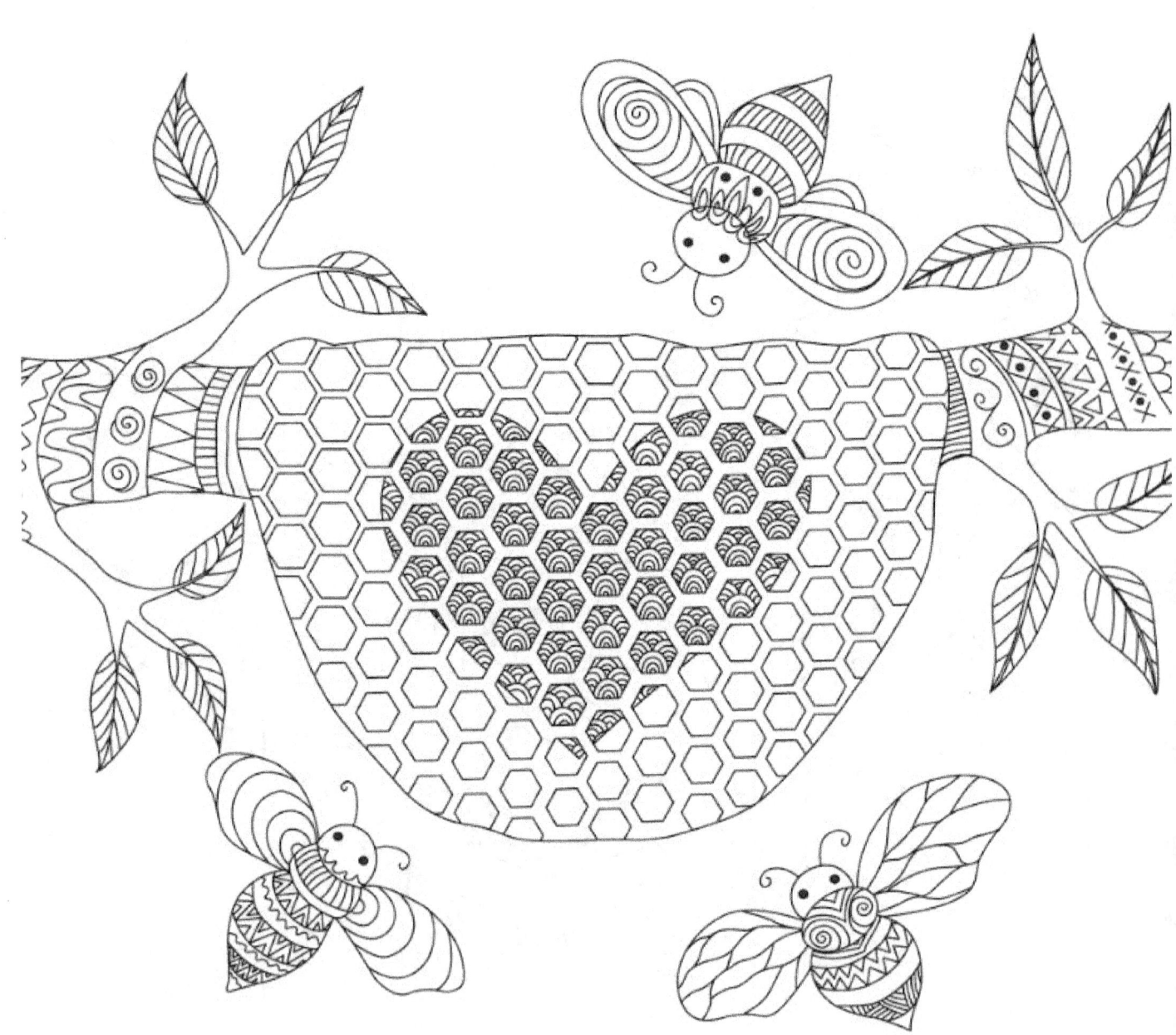

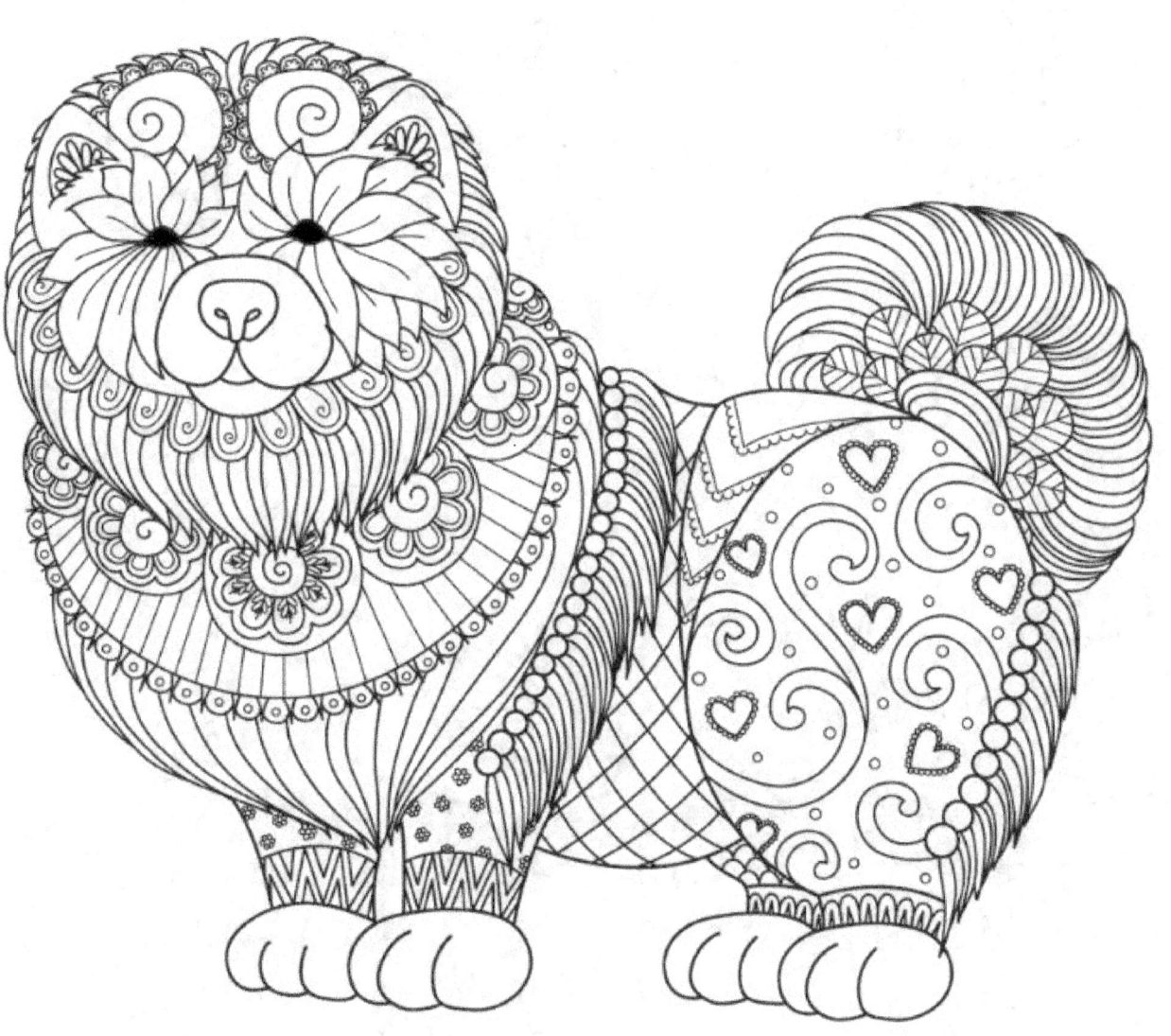

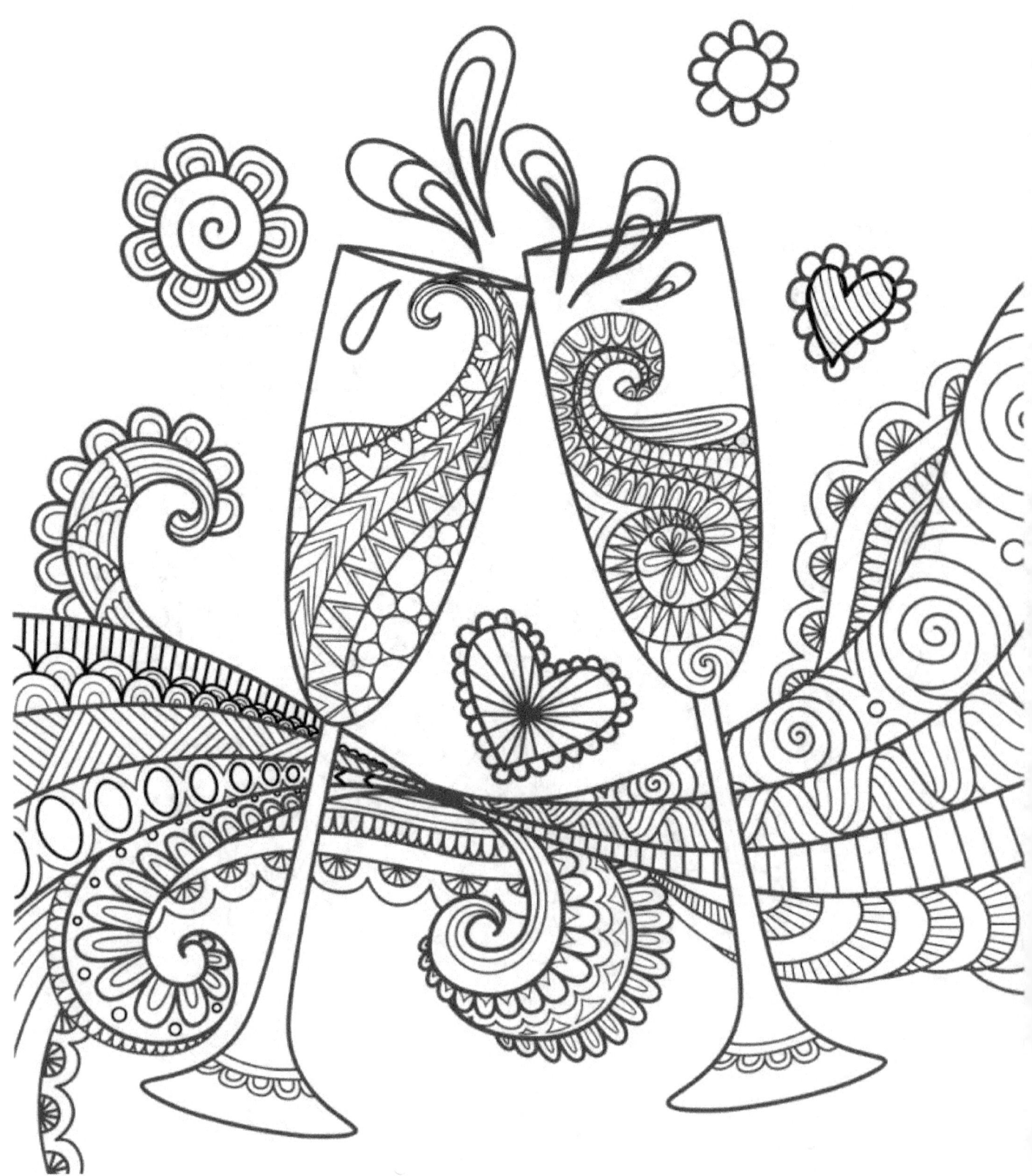

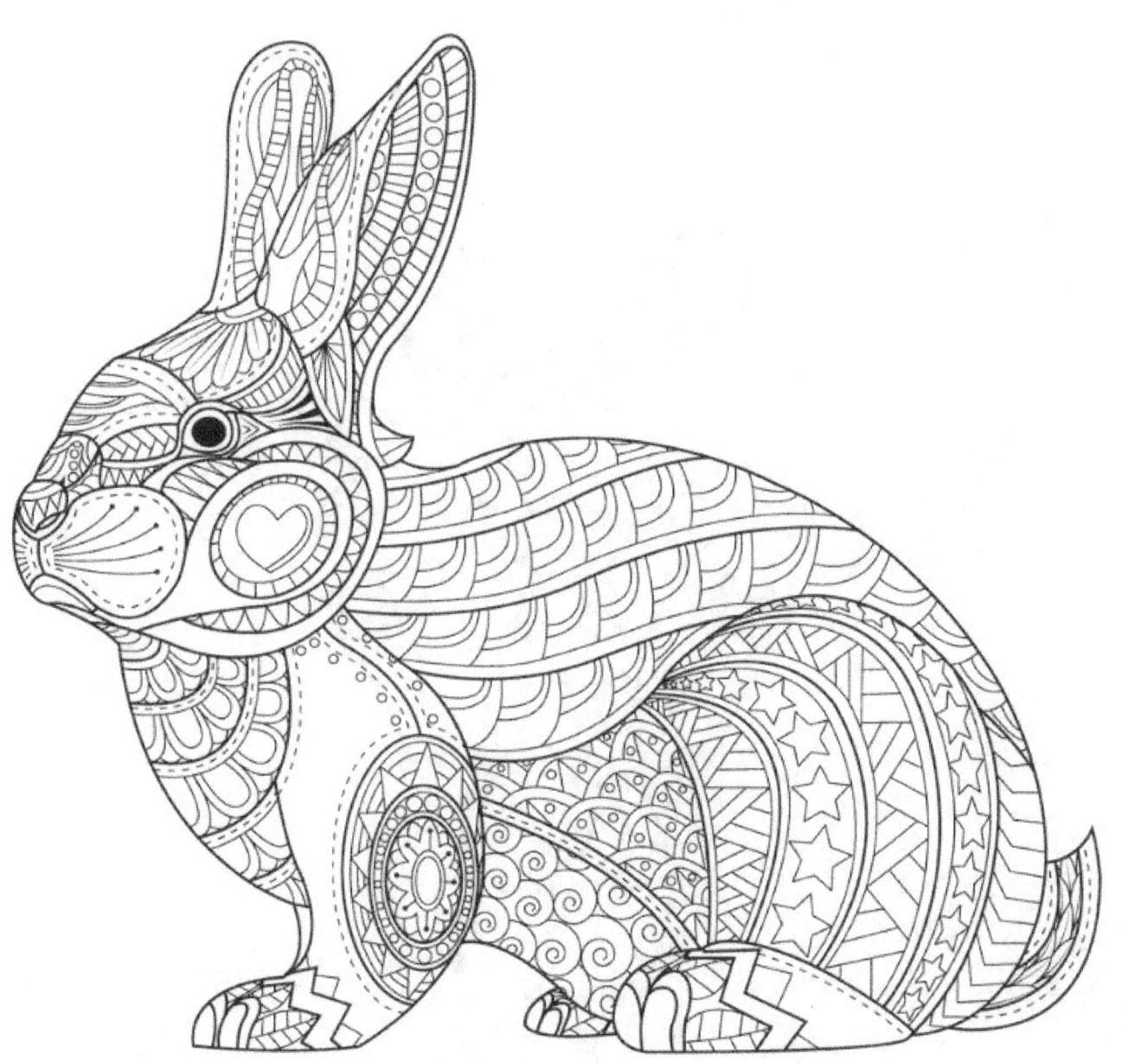

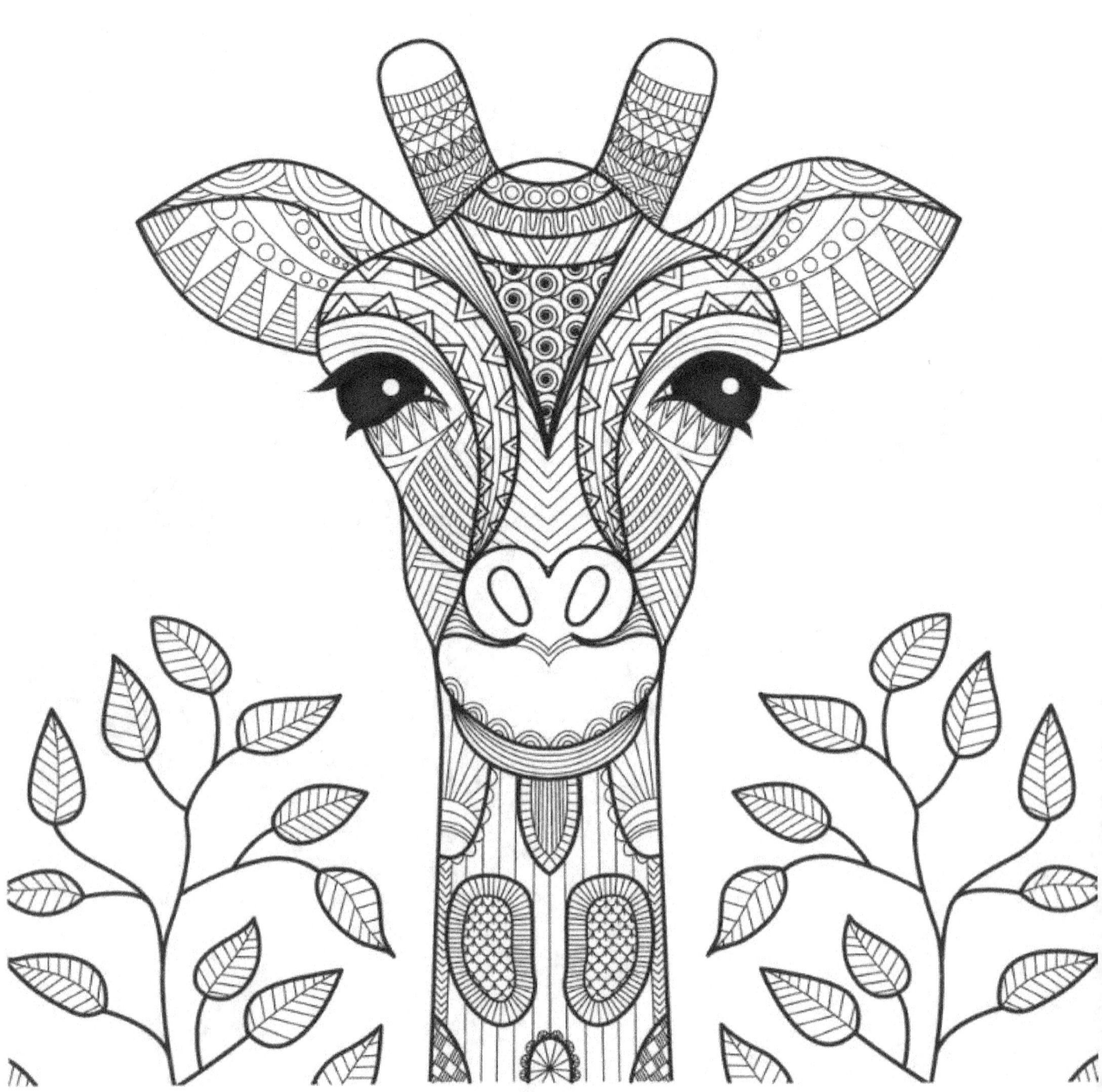

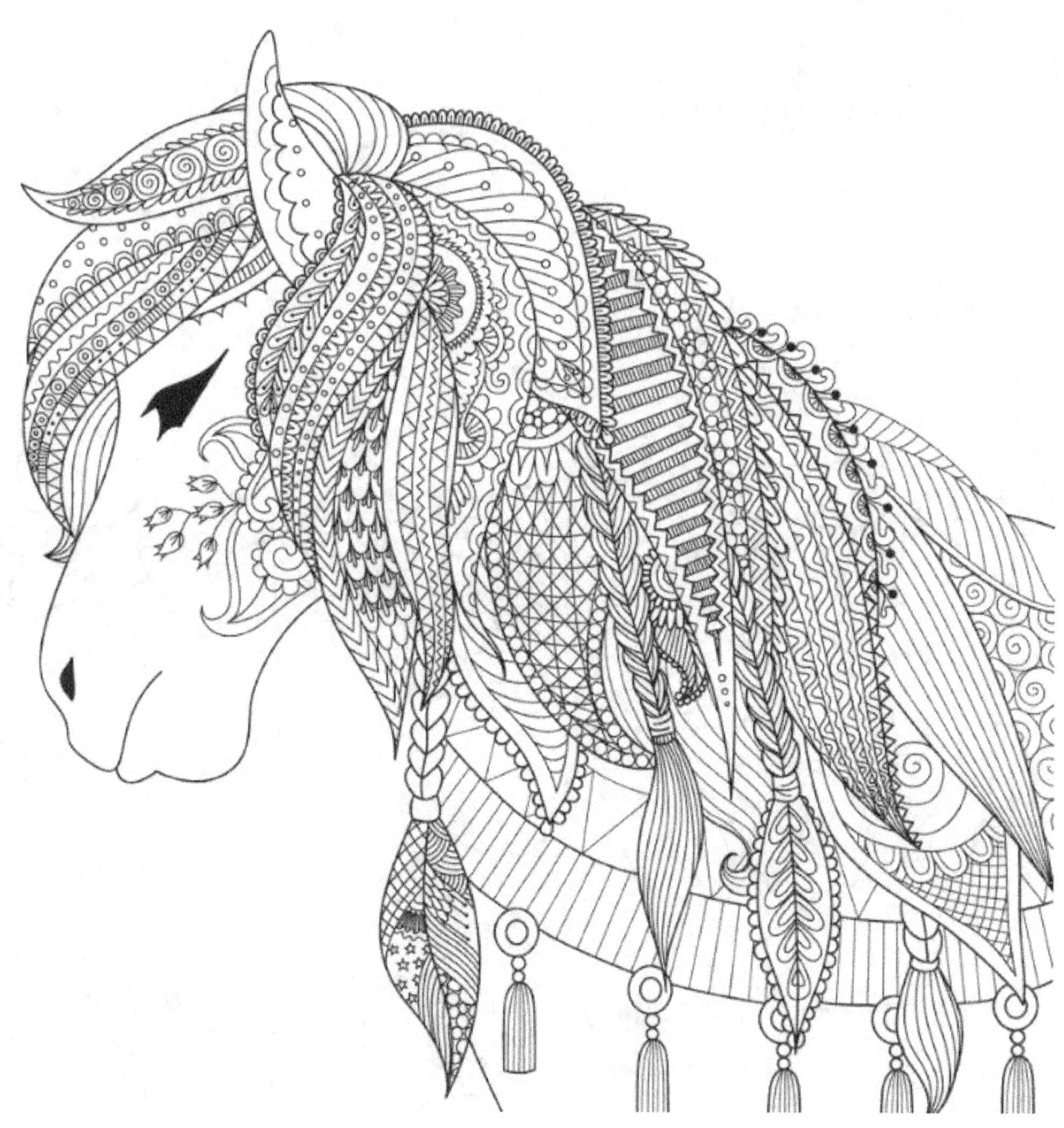

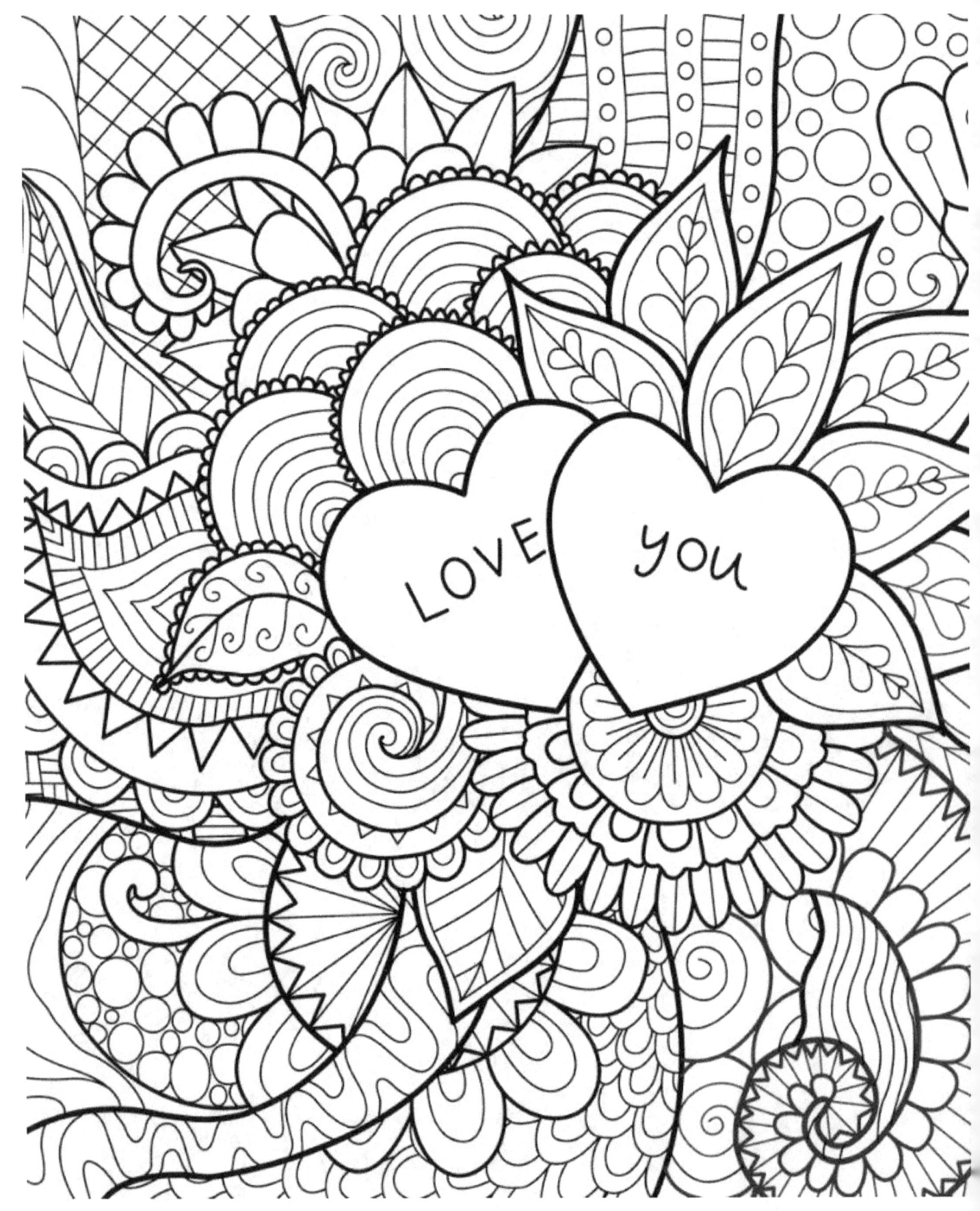

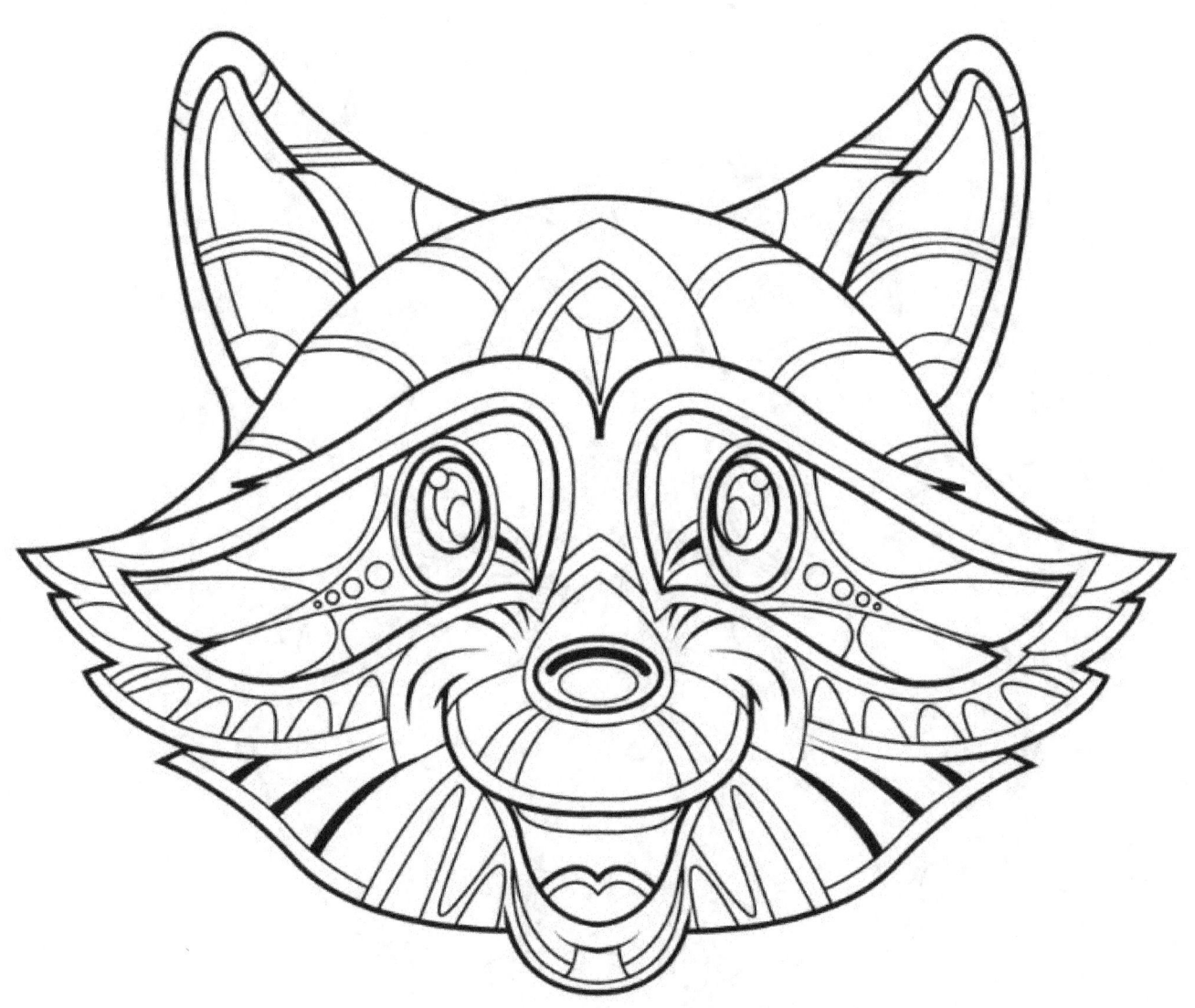

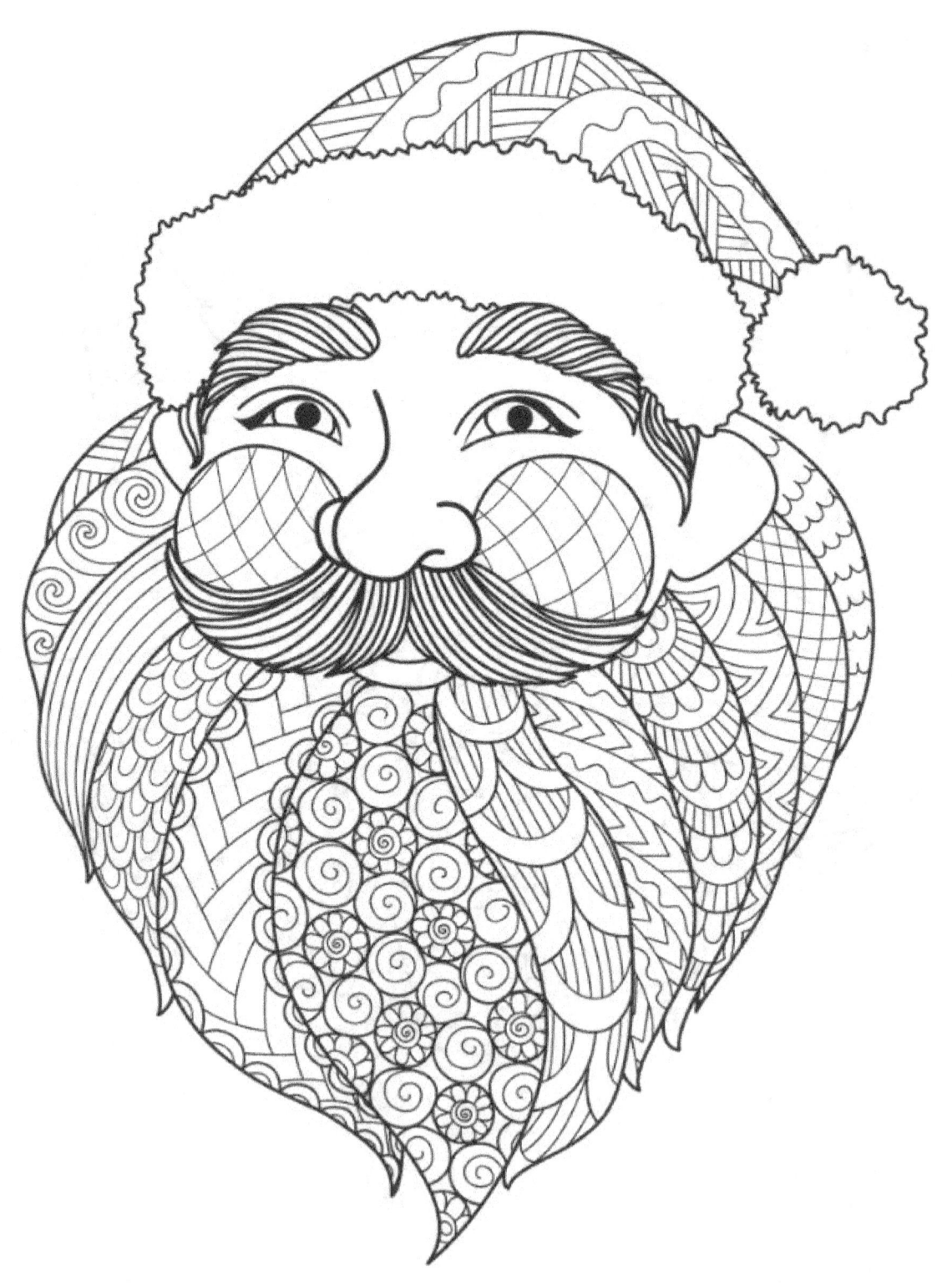

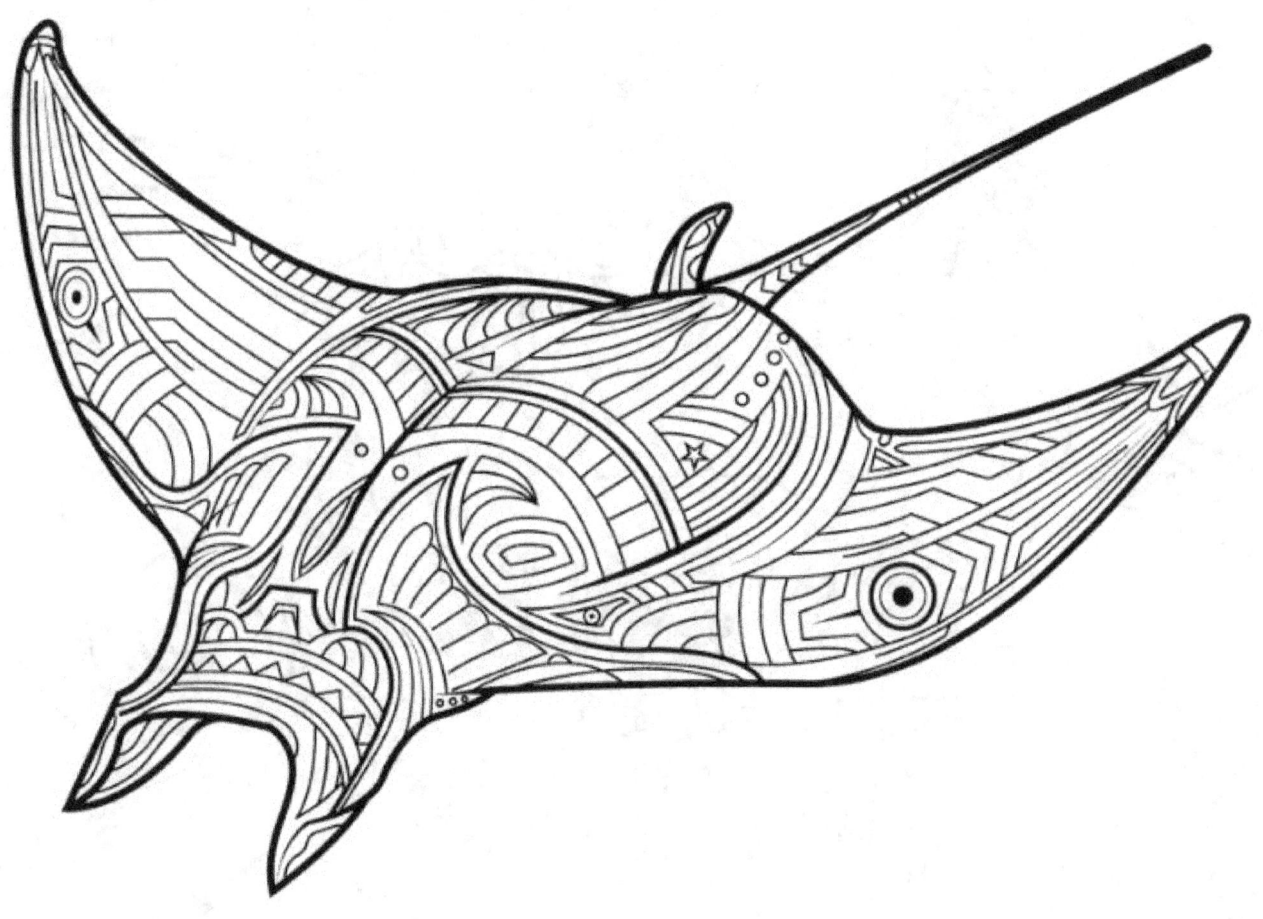

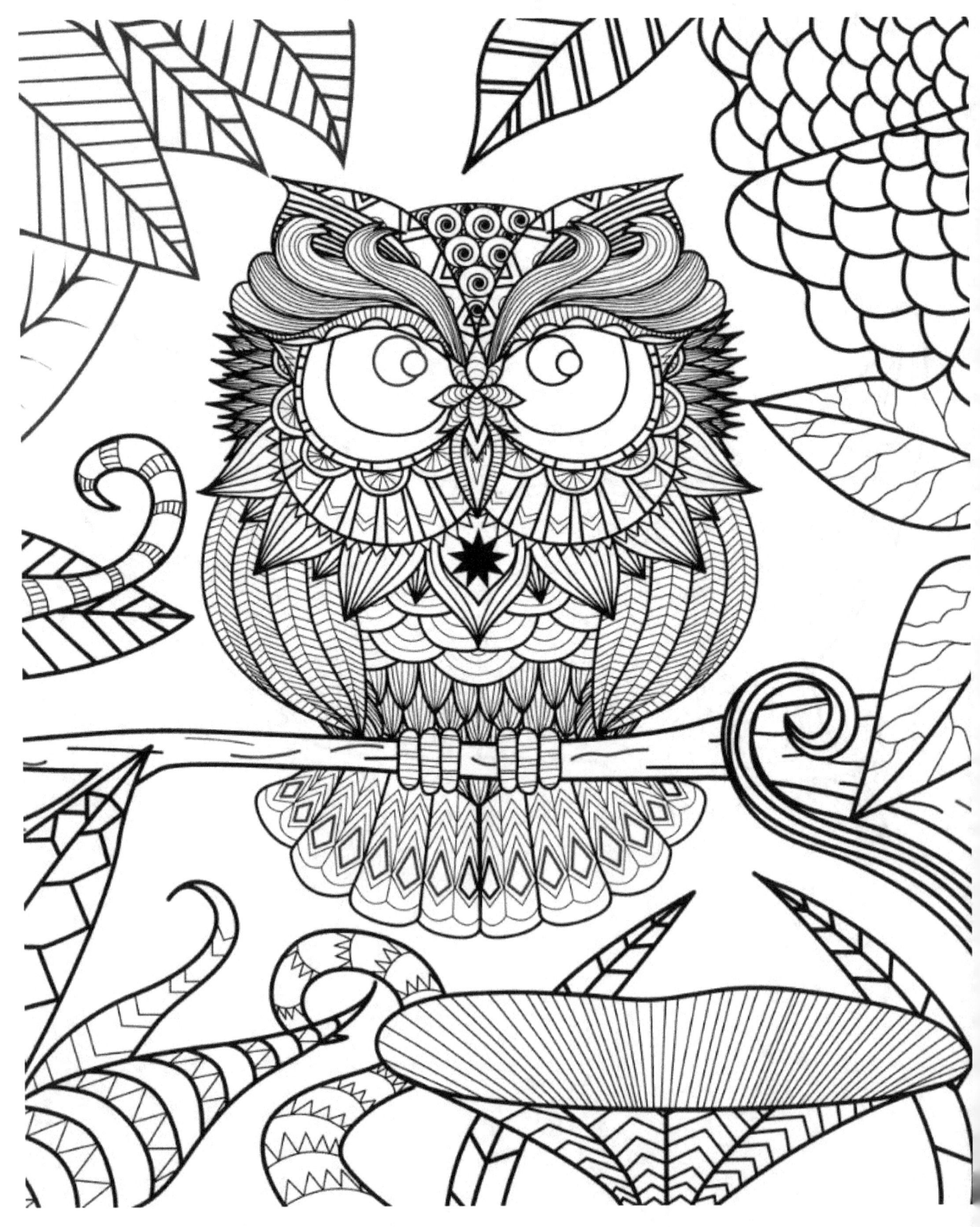

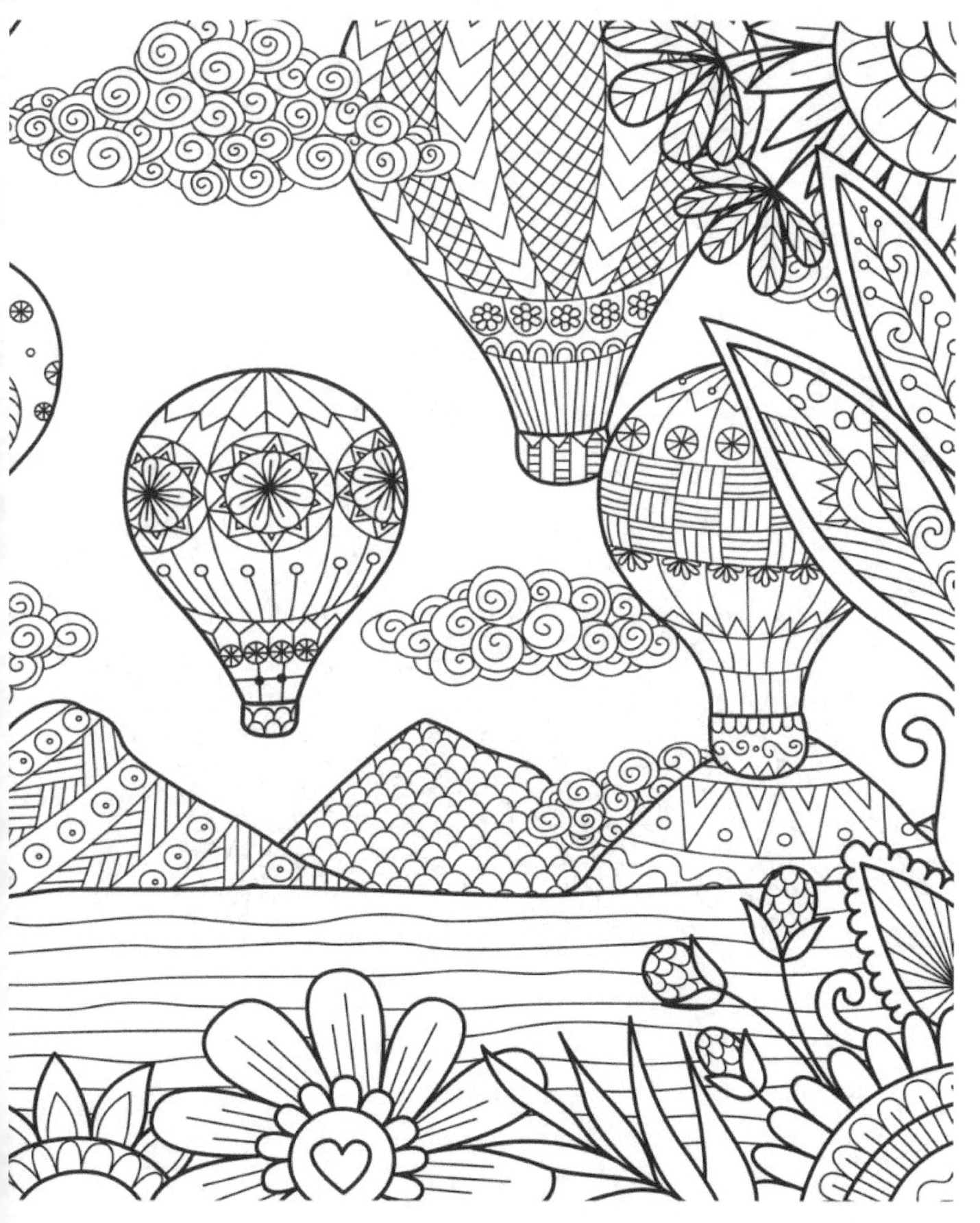

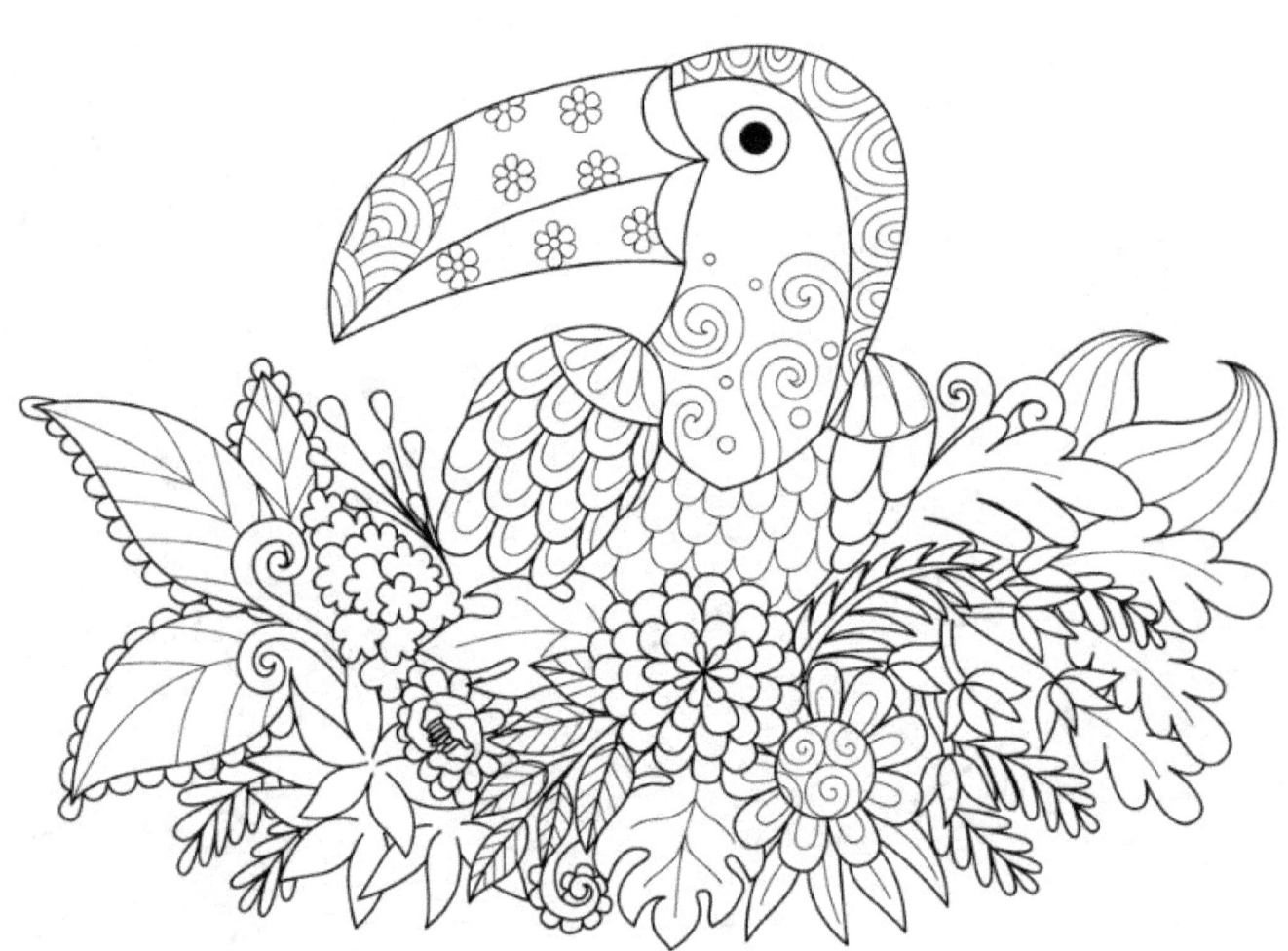

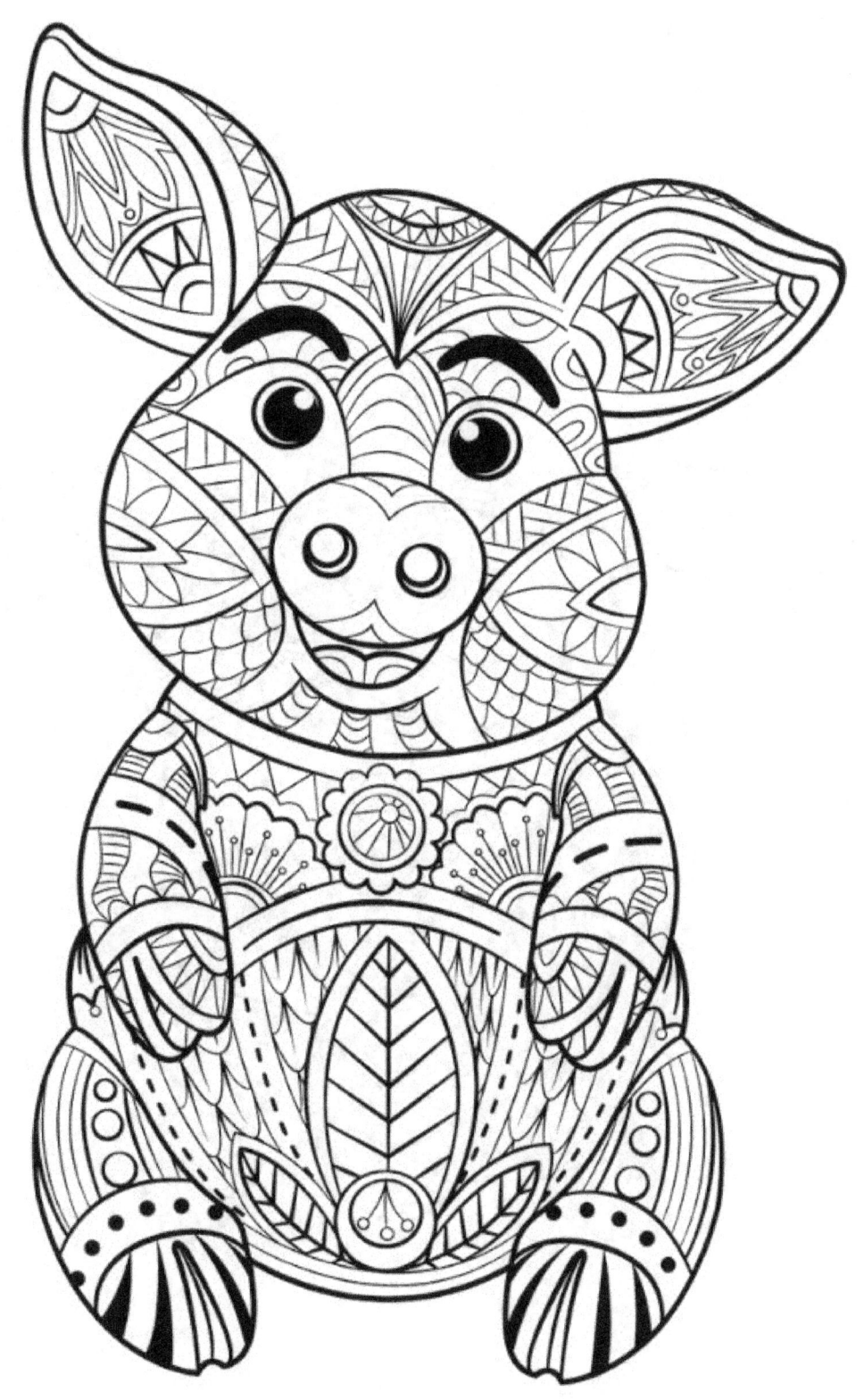

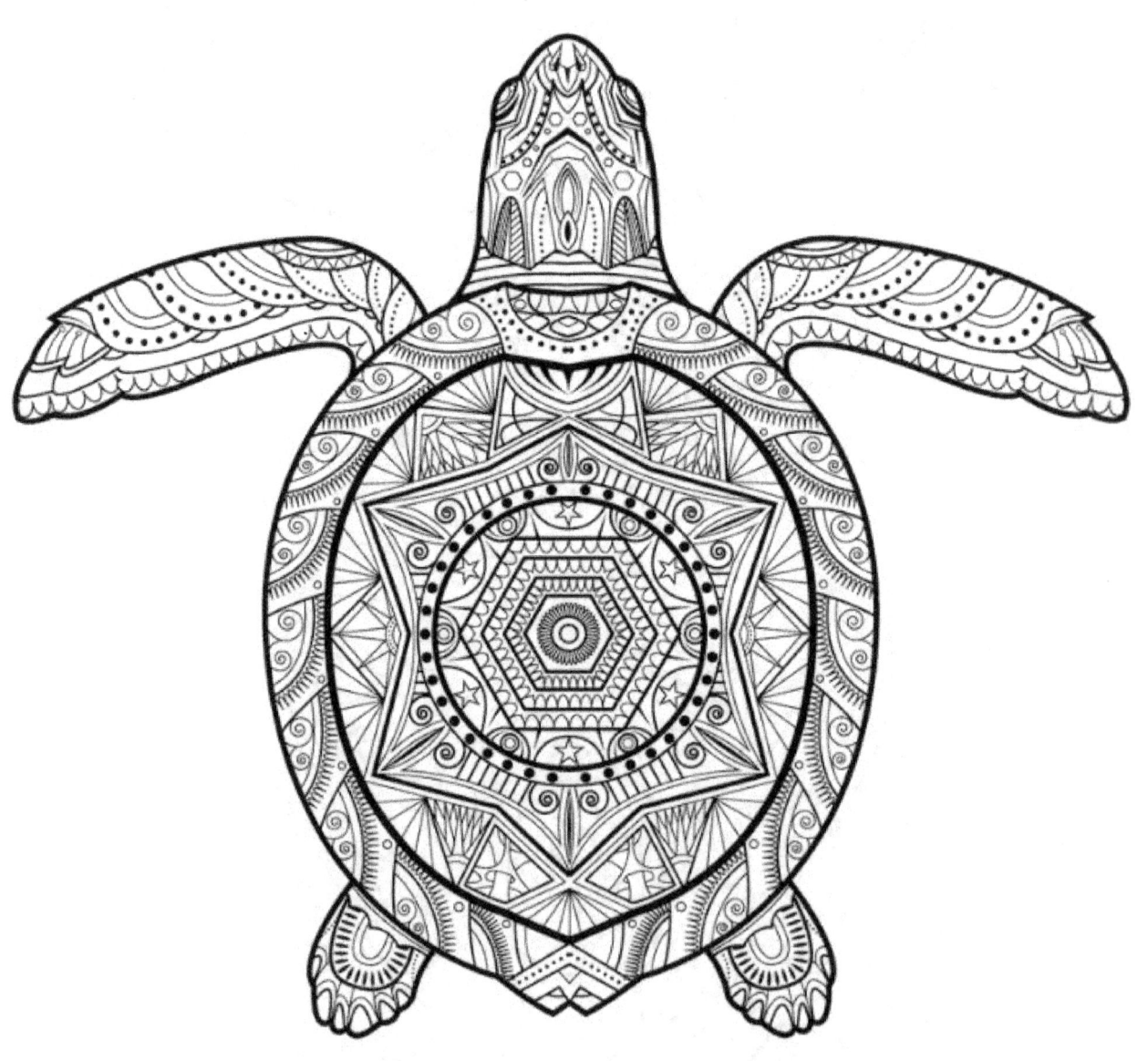

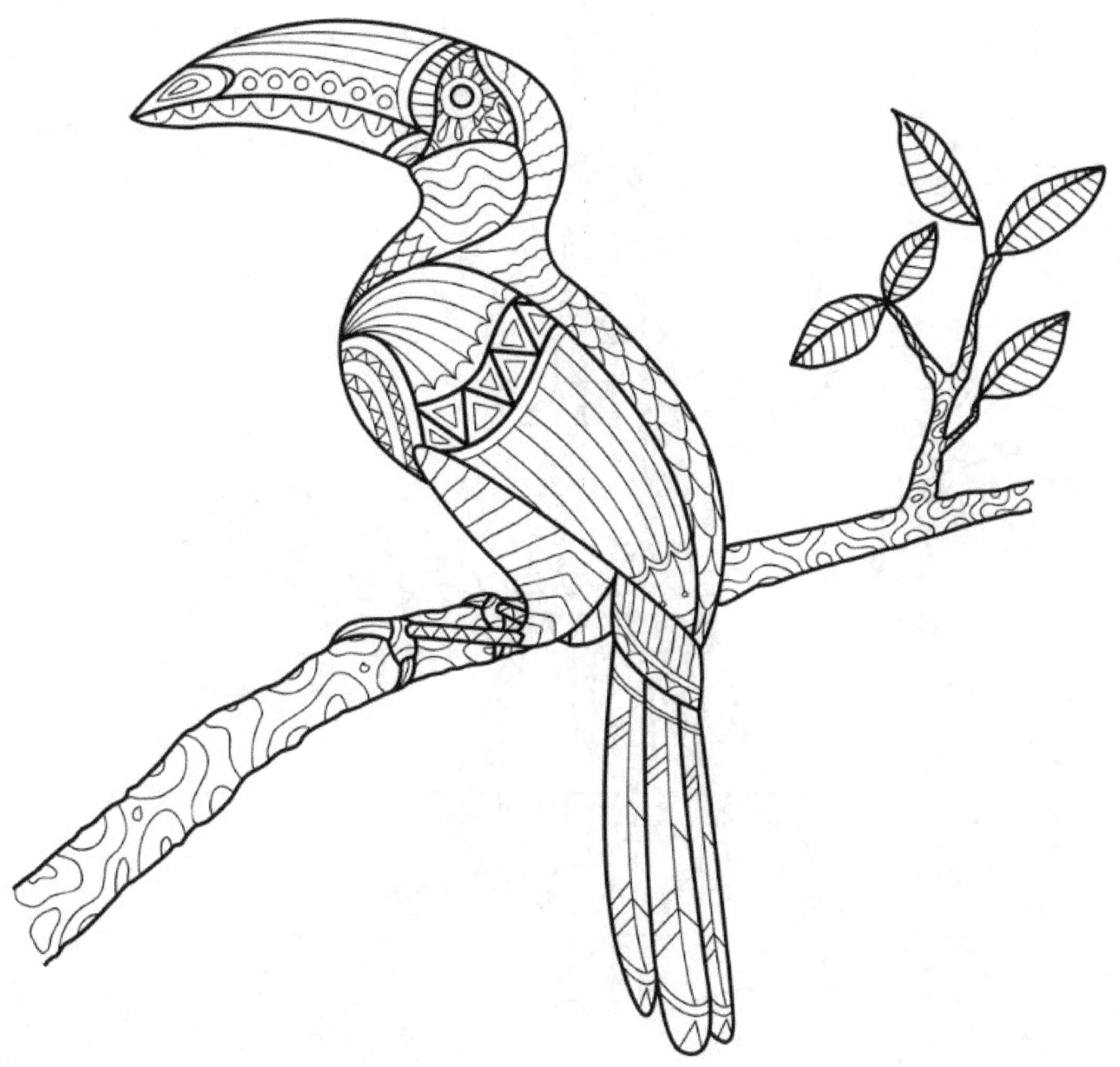

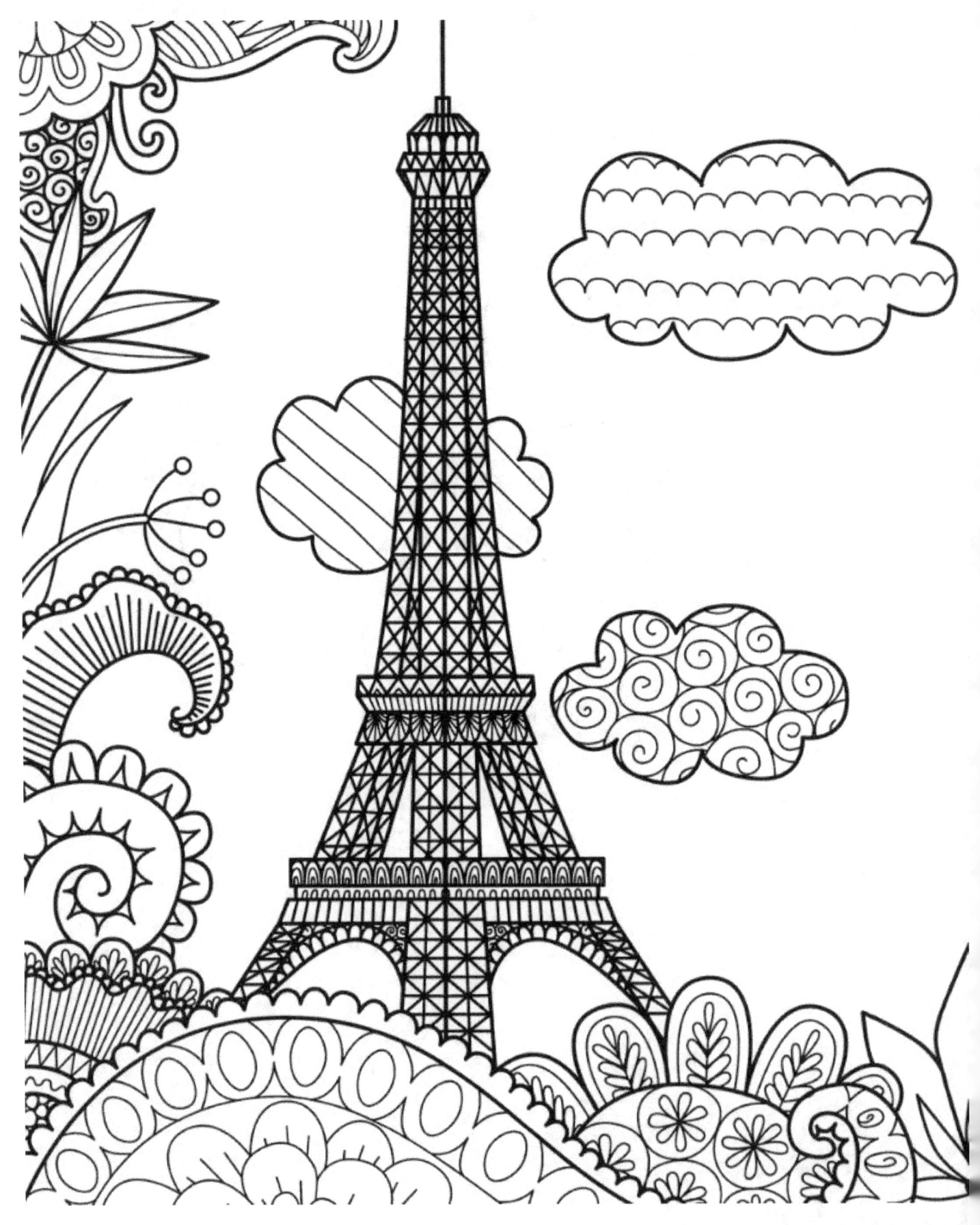

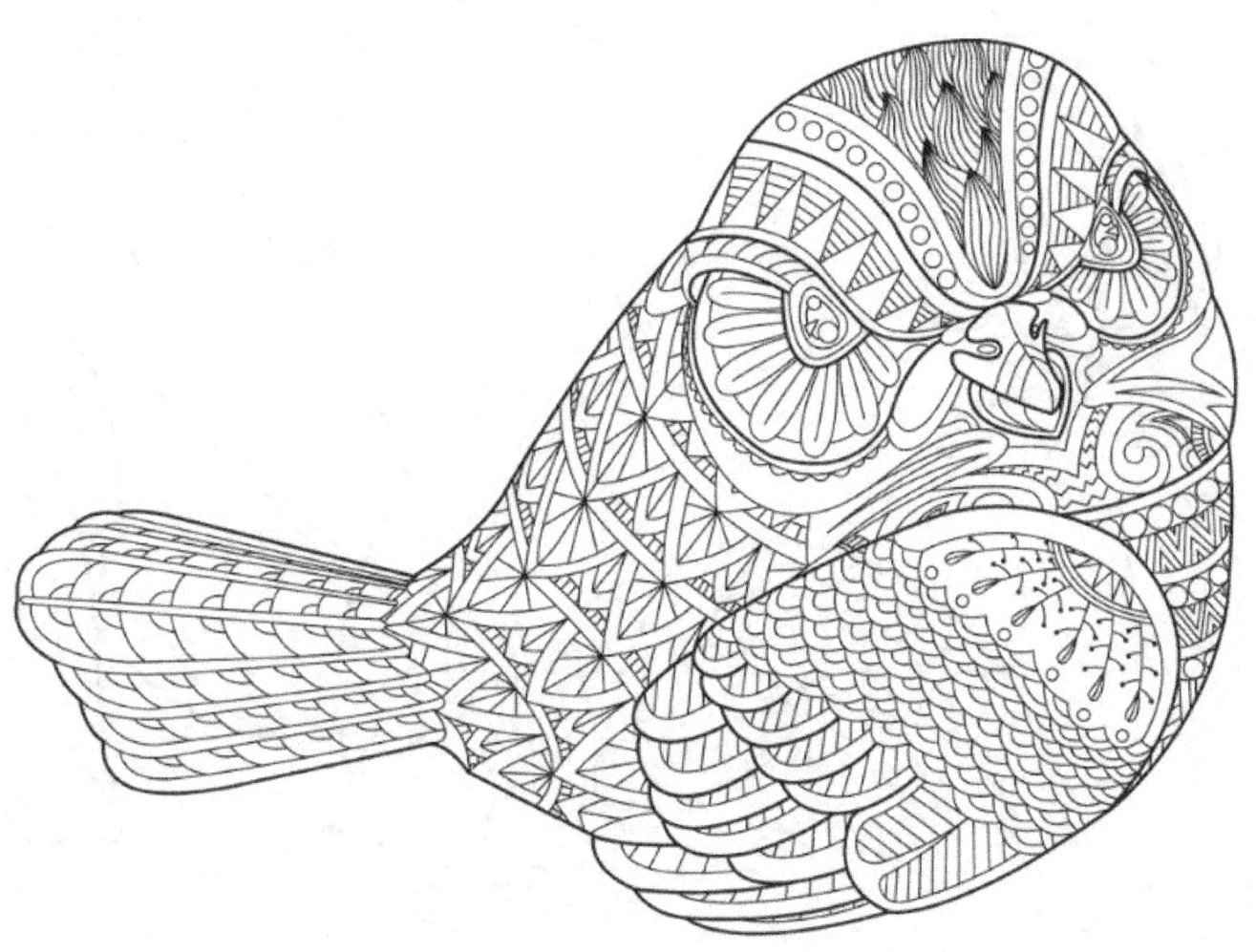

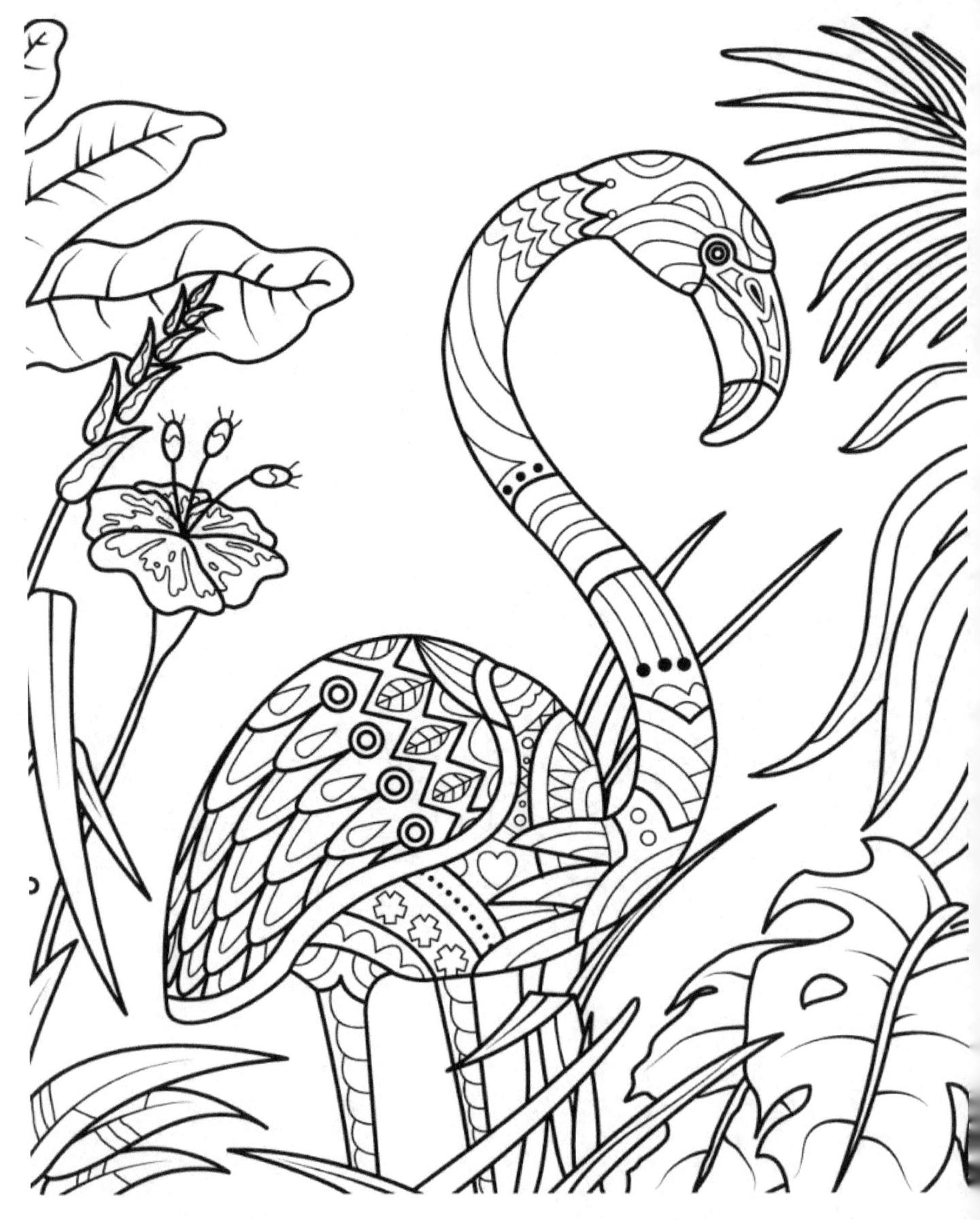

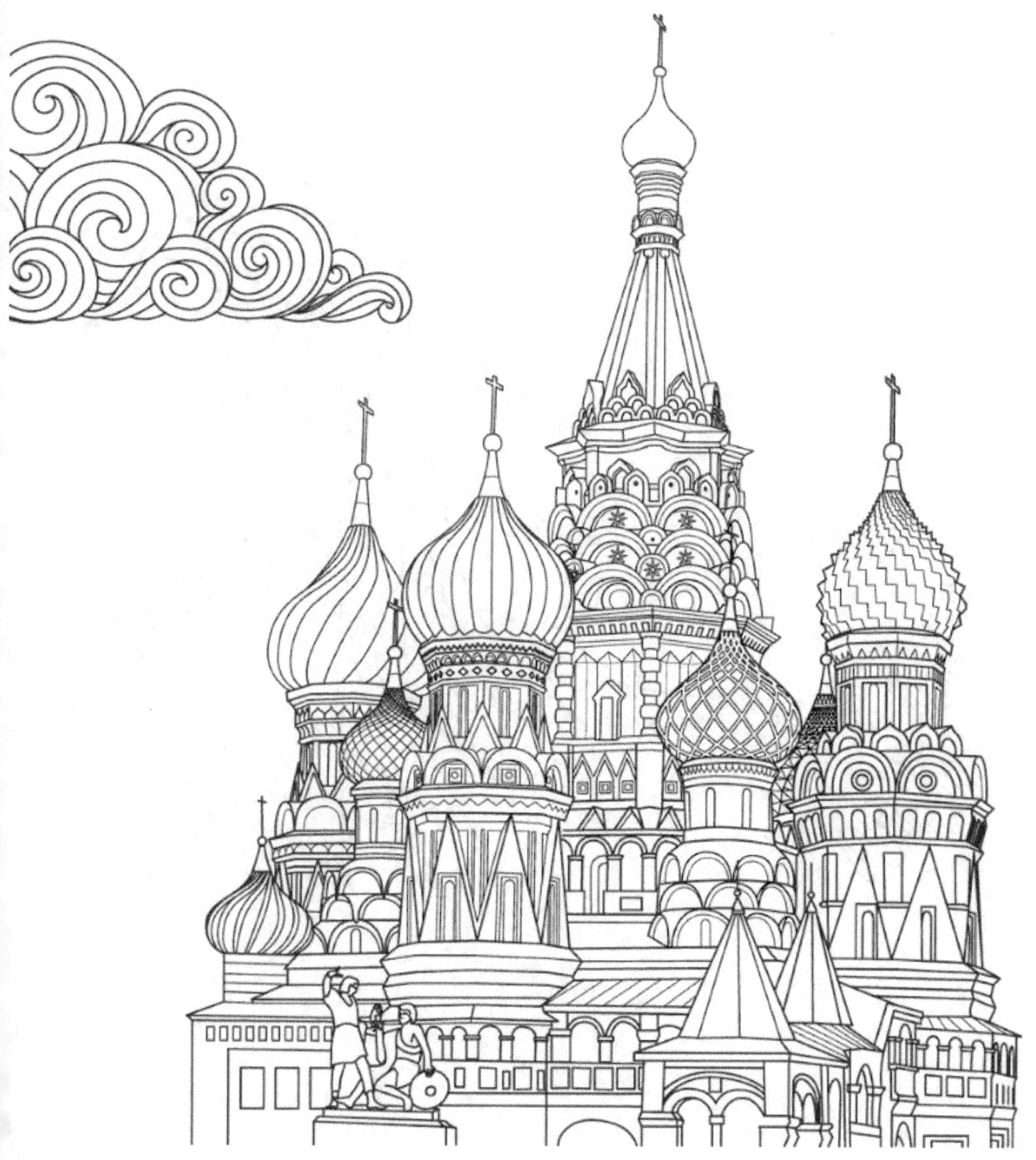

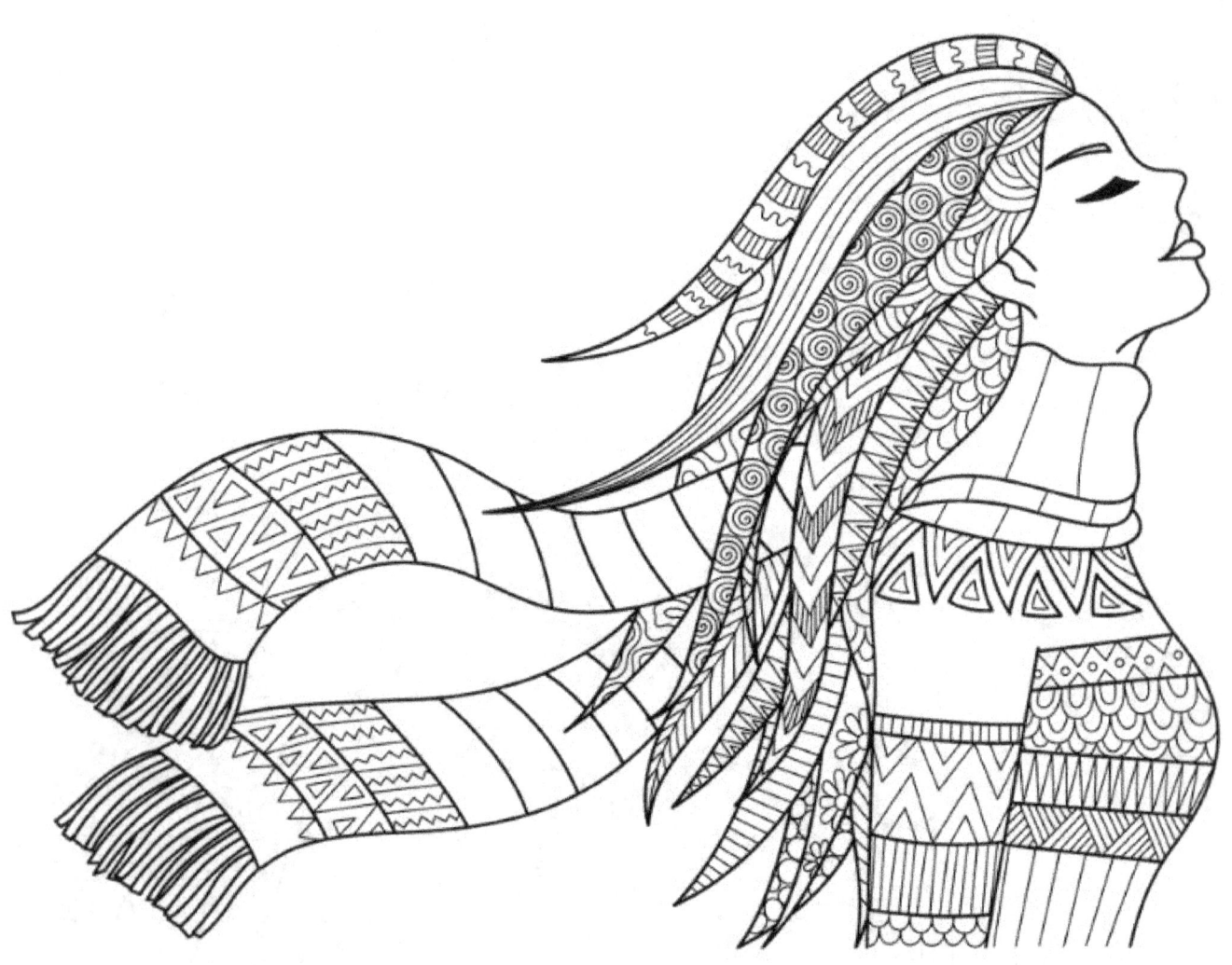

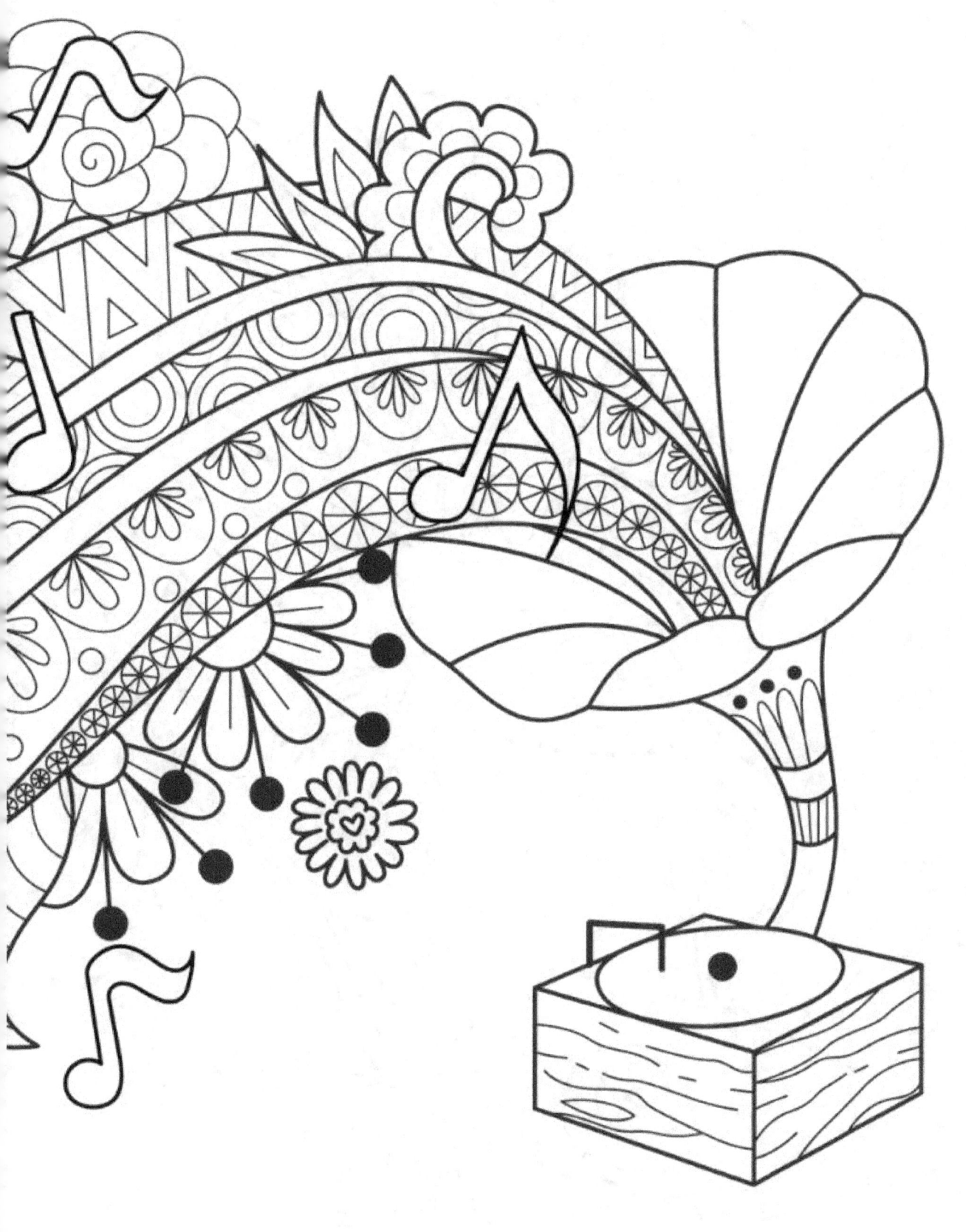

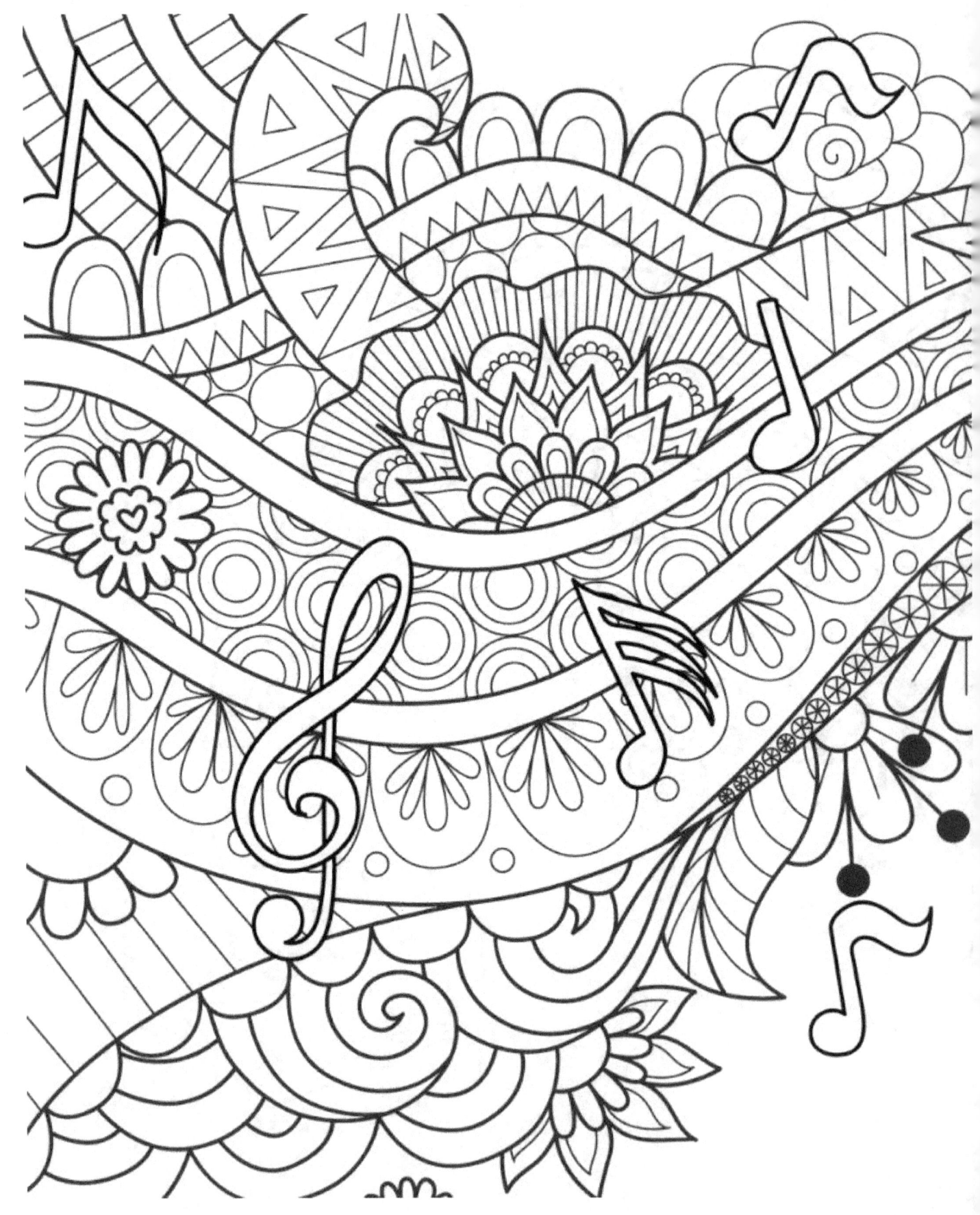

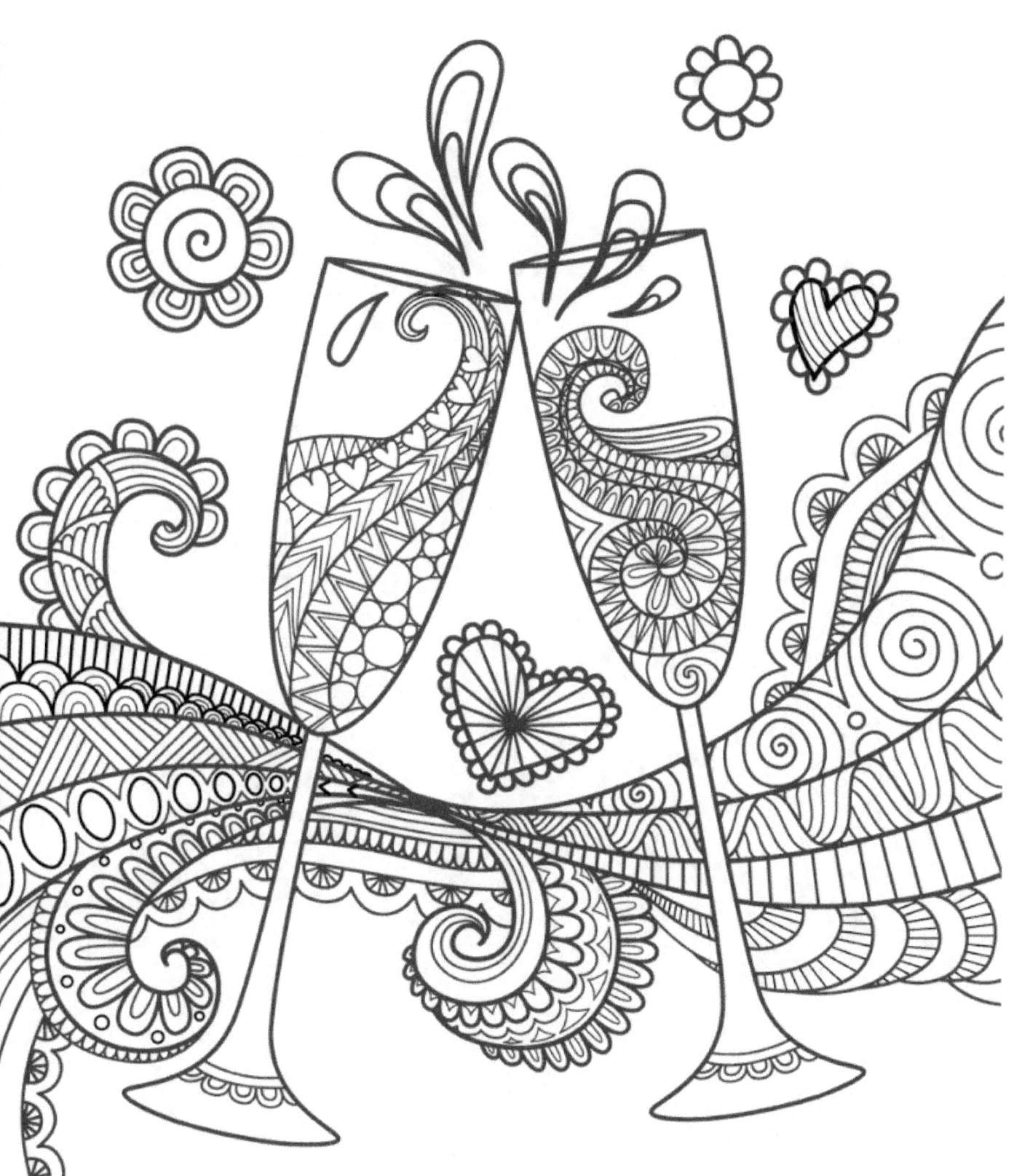

www.ingramcontent.com/pod-product-compliance
Lightning Source LLC
Chambersburg PA
CBHW081024170526
45158CB00010B/3154